NATUREBIRTH

Danaë Brook was born in England. The mother of three children herself, she runs classes in preparation for conscious birth. Having won a *Vogue* talents competition she became a feature writer for the *Daily Express* and now contributes articles to a wide variety of newspapers and magazines, as well as broadcasting on radio and television. Danaë Brook lives in London.

D1471675

Naturebirth

PREPARING FOR NATURAL BIRTH IN AN AGE
OF TECHNOLOGY

Danaë Brook

Foreword by
PETER J. HUNTINGFORD

PENGUIN BOOKS

Penguin Books Ltd, Harmondsworth, Middlesex, England
Penguin Books, 625 Madison Avenue, New York, New York 10022, U.S.A.
Penguin Books Australia Ltd, Ringwood, Victoria, Australia
Penguin Books Canada Ltd, 2801 John Street, Markham, Ontario, Canada L3R 1B4
Penguin Books (N.Z.) Ltd, 182–190 Wairau Road, Auckland 10, New Zealand

—

Published simultaneously by Penguin Books and William Heinemann 1976
Reprinted 1979

—

Copyright © Danaë Brook 1976
Illustrations and charts copyright © Danaë Brook and A. T. Mann, 1976
All rights reserved

—

Figure drawings by Maureen Duff

—

Made and printed in Great Britain by
Richard Clay (The Chaucer Press) Ltd, Bungay, Suffolk
Set in Monotype Times

For John with love

John is my husband and my lover. Since he has been my mainstay and sanity through the cathartic experiences of having babies and writing a book, the dedication of *Naturebirth* is first to him. Without his perception, I would not have seen; without his patience, I would not have persevered; without his strength, I would never have finished this book, which is the laying down of our return to nature having understood the magic of childbirth.

I have also to thank my three sons, Peter, Orion and Liam, for keeping me constantly in touch with the truth I learned through them; and my mother for teaching me the validity of instinct and the power of family love.

Author's Note:

I have chosen to describe the embryo and fetus, in other words, the unborn child, as 'he' for the very personal reason that my babies have all been boys, so I inevitably relate to that memory. I feel it is really important to approach the unborn and the newly born as a real person, not some sexless 'it' that sounds like a robot. Please take it as understood that I mean 'he' or 'she', 'him' or 'her', but it is simply too long-winded to write that every time . . .

Contents

Contents

Foreword

Naturebirth is not another cult of childbirth. It does not seek to replace current methods. Danaë Brook is a pragmatist, who acknowledges that destruction of the established norms achieves little unless there are alternatives to replace them. She also realizes that the development of revolutionary ideas can produce just as much limitation of freedom as the order that provoked the revolt.

Danaë Brook seeks to make women spiritually self-reliant in childbirth despite the drive of modern obstetric practice to make women conform. She invites women to promote change by asking questions—and she asks some good questions. Questions, which obstetricians and midwives should listen to, and learn from the answers. Why do men dominate the conduct of childbearing? Why are women humiliated by the rituals of enemas, pubic shaves, induction of labour and episiotomy? Why should we sacrifice the humane treatment of women as individuals to the mechanized anonymous safety of our impersonal ante-natal clinics and labour wards? Why should physical safety be divorced from the achievement of emotional satisfaction?

No doubt many obstetricians and midwives will criticize *Naturebirth* quite severely, but few women will do so. Danaë Brook speaks as a woman to women out of her own experiences. Such spoken thoughts are just as valid and helpful to others about to have the same experience as a wealth of profound scientific knowledge.

Danaë Brook has provided me as a male obstetrician with knowledge and insight that I did not have before reading the book. I may find it difficult from my orthodox medical background to accept her references to homoeopathy and astrology, but her open-minded tolerance of their contribution makes me want to do the same. She offers a challenge to the medical profession, inviting them to change their attitudes. Her book, I am sure, will encourage women. It will enable them to rely on their innate practical common sense, and above all on themselves as women seeking fulfilment in childbirth.

PETER J. HUNTINGFORD
London, February 1976.

> 'The fundamental conception of sympathetic magic is identical with that of modern science; underlying the whole system is a faith, implicit but real and firm, in the order and uniformity of nature.'
>
> J. G. FRAZER
> *The Golden Bough*

I found in my life that I had lost touch with the idea of magic I knew as a child and was rapidly losing touch with nature. Giving birth spun me full circle and brought me back to the essence of things, to see the establishing of man's unity with nature as magic.

Naturebirth is my heart and soul on paper. I learned something which changed my whole life, when I gave birth consciously, sharing the experience with my lover. The book that follows is an explanation of this experience, but it is also a tool for you, a guide, a synthesizing of all the information I have gathered over the past few years, in case some of the information might affect positively the event of birth for people who might not otherwise be aware of how powerful the experience can be.

The facts of birth are important. But I have found that evidence conflicts, information changes, sources vary, viewpoints vacillate and within the medical profession itself methods and theories contradict. Instinct is vitally important. This is an unchanging truth. Relying on yourself, being aware of your inner rhythms, provides a security which remains constant in the turbulent conditions of pregnancy and birth today. Hopefully this book of words may bridge the gap between instinct and scientific research for those who recognize the need for such a bridge.

Naturebirth

I see men and women floundering in the contradictions of their civilization, searching for alternatives to present life. Birth is a beginning. I believe if we prepare ourselves to understand the nature of birth better than our twentieth-century conditioning allows, and are more aware of life as it is occurring, the experience will bring greater fulfilment to women, greater depth to the union of man and woman, greater stability to the family, a sounder foundation for living.

This is how it happened for me.

A Personal Introduction

I start with my own story, because I know it best. I write of the woman who introduced me to prepared childbirth, because I believe we can all teach each other, and the process of learning and teaching is a process of exchange that is both subtle and vital to the full experience of natural childbirth, Naturebirth. Pregnancy causes people, especially women, to react and relate more subjectively than they do normally, however militant an armour of 'liberation' they may wear in their unpregnant daily lives—and it is far easier to compare experiences with other people than grasp the complex language of specialists. I am not an expert, only a woman experienced in a particular field of knowledge in that I have borne three children and had the benefit of advice from a good teacher. Rather than claim expertise I would just say, look, I have learned something about life from birth. There's something in it for you too. But to learn, you must raise questions and challenge many accepted assumptions.

In certain ways I am a feminist. I believe in the equality of opportunities for men and women and will fight for that. But I also believe we can extend the boundaries of feminism into motherhood. And should. I do not believe that freeing ourselves from the restriction and prejudice of a society based on discrimination and institutions should mean that we lose sight of our essential nature, whether male or female. To me liberation means integration and balance, not schisms and labels, and one set of rules and roles exchanged for another. As a woman, it means finding that balance in being a mother as well as in being a single woman, because at one time or other most of us are faced with the question of whether or not we

3

become mothers, and why. At the height of my own chaotic revolution, I discovered that to call myself a revolutionary was dishonest unless I could make the principles of honesty, freedom, communication and awareness work within my own family. When I became pregnant with my second son, I realized that the place to begin was birth.

My first son, Peter, was born when I was very young, unprepared and alone. The experience was terrifying and I wanted never to repeat it. My second son, Orion, was born after a lonely pregnancy during the break-up of a marriage, but after preparing myself his birth was pure elation. My third son, Liam, was born in a burst of sunlight after a pregnancy spent getting ready for his birth in close communion with my lover, the father of my child. It was after this I realized I had something to tell.

There is no such thing as a textbook pregnancy or labour, so there cannot be an absolute blueprint for either, simply suggestions and information, because that is every parent's right. There is no perfect labour, so it would be a pointless goal. But there is sensitivity, awareness, sense—and there can be a blueprint by which you can prepare yourselves with these qualities, for giving birth. Preparation is a guidance. It is about sustaining courage in the face of the unexpected, which needs a particular kind of inner strength, rooted in confidence and knowledge; and it is about dealing with pain through relaxation. It is for men and women together and for women alone; women who are working, who are single, who are old and young, happy and sad, brave and frightened, resentful and willing. It is for heterosexuals and homosexuals and bisexuals, for freaks and family people alike, because birth is simultaneously the most sensitive and most dangerous moment in the life of every one of us. Giving birth requires a total commitment to be experienced on every level; it demands of us the highest we can give in physical, emotional and spiritual energy. Not everyone is ready to give this. To me and my husband, accepting that conditions of birth are likely to affect future life meant that we felt obliged to see if we could do something about easing birth for our own children. For the logical sequence must be that a child cannot be born without physical and possibly psychological distress to a woman who is in a physically or psychologically distressed state. We prepared to develop awareness and take action.

In the event our vital discovery was that knowing ourselves and coming to grips with what was happening in my body gave us physical and emotional strength. It also equipped us to deal with medical institutions and establishments that are not in the habit of questioning their methods of birth. Everyone has the right to question and the right to know. This book is for those who want to know.

*   *   *

It begins with the birth of Orion, my middle son, because this was the point of change. This was the first birth I prepared for. This preparation changed my attitude to birth from negative to positive. During the first seven months Orion was inside me, I was trying to handle, as coolly as possible, the dissolution of a ten-year marriage to the father of my eldest son, Peter, and the child I was expecting, Orion. I had loved my husband, but found I couldn't live with him. He was the father of this new child, but didn't want to be. I didn't know if I could be a mother alone, but I did know I had to try. Although I had met the man I was later to live with and eventually marry, it was not the time to call for his help. It was the time to find strength within myself.

About four weeks before the child was born, I met a woman called Sara Harrison who told me she could guide me through the birth so that it was not the horror I remembered from having my first child. She told me preparation could transform the experience. Perhaps unusually, I didn't know there were places where you could learn the various forms of natural childbirth, and neither doctor nor hospital had pointed me in that direction. I didn't believe Sara when she said it was within my power to change the experience of birth, but I wanted it to be true. So I sat with her through winter mornings in a room full of cushions, learning strange breathing exercises, going back through the memory of that previous birth. Like an exorcism perhaps. Spilling it out. The swamping contractions, the tidal wave, the fear that you will never get through which makes you fight your own body and the incredible forces at work, instead of allowing it all to happen so that giving birth becomes like making love and in nine months we move from orgasm to orgasm.

Sara and I first met in an October London that shook a snakeskin of marmalade leaves along the street from my house to hers. When she opened the door to me the first time my stomach popped through first and caught her by surprise.

5

'Didn't know you were that far on,' she smiled at me.

'Got in a panic,' I said sheepishly. 'I looked at it in the bath and suddenly realized I was going to have a baby in less than a month and I remembered I wanted to die the last time.'

Her handshake was firm and cool and drew me inside.

'It's okay,' she said. 'There are a few things you can do to sort through those feelings.'

So she took me on. Her first pupil in England.

Sara had been living in California for several years, helping to prepare women for birth. When in London she went through a teachers' training course at the National Childbirth Trust which qualified her to give ante-natal preparation classes. The Trust itself is an organization which aims to educate women to have their babies 'happily and free from fear'. Their concern is to make sure that as much information is made available to pregnant women as possible.

'Happily and free from fear', to Sara, meant as naturally as possible. She worked out a way of teaching women to relax enough to deal with the enormous sensations of birth, using fewer drugs and greater self-awareness than was generally encouraged by the medical profession. It seemed labour could actually become less painful through a woman's willingness to flow with the physical changes in her body instead of reacting against them. She discovered that for a woman to manage her own labour she needed the benefit of a full physical, intellectual and emotional preparation, part of which was a specific breathing technique. It was this preparation she wanted to give to me.

I was ready. Her personal apprenticeship to the profession of easing childbirth was wide enough to impress me without being intimidating. And I, like many other women, am intimidated by authoritarian figures. The most important thing was that Sara was a mother, she had experienced giving birth, she could talk and explain as much from her own experience of having children, as from being taught how to teach. It gave my own learning process a sense of immediacy. She had developed her personal knowledge into a kind of therapeutic preparation which combined the ideas of relaxation, the principles of Yoga exercises to which correct breathing is intrinsic, Wilhelm Reich's theories on freeing sexual energy by 'unblocking' tense areas of the body, current information on medical techniques and the breathing method propounded by the National Childbirth Trust and most natural childbirth organizations, that of 'psychoprophylaxis'—or 'mental-prevention' as it translates literally. Her special gift lay in a particular ability to spice the mixture by encouraging people to open up and talk about themselves with complete honesty.

Psychoprophylaxis was first developed by the Russians, who used it as a distraction technique to cope with stress, especially in labour. The entire teaching is complex, but, put simply, it means that the mind can prevent the body's extreme discomfort from stress. It has been used and interpreted by many, the best known of them being the French doctors, Fernand Lamaze and Pierre Vellay. Each teacher following each school of thought in turn develops the fundamental idea in his or her own way of putting it across. Sara's way appealed to me because there was so little formality, yet such broad scope for understanding and discussion. She admitted that pregnancy alters many facets of the lives involved and beginning from there, attempted to prepare men and women both physically and mentally, without ducking the crucial issues. No subject was taboo. No fear too grotesque to examine. No hope too wild to give rein to. I think that one of the most serious limitations of modern obstetrics is that childbirth, or the state of being pregnant, is viewed as an affliction of the belly for which only the lower half of the body is treated. Sara's preparation was for the whole being. She has continued to develop her own techniques of teaching in the West of England, where she has since settled. Clearly I write from my personal experience of her as a woman, and of her work. This book of preparation is my interpretation of the way she taught me then and my exploration of the things I learned.

In that light-footed swelling-bellied autumn of 1970 I was the first woman to ask her help since she had left California to set up home in London. The two of us faced the reality of a new labour and a new child. I didn't feel like a pupil because she didn't come on like a teacher. It was just like talking to an intimate friend. Her silence persuasive, her comments wry, funny, and understanding—relating her own experiences to mine, so that I didn't feel alone.

'Now you have a fresh start,' she told me. 'It's a new pregnancy, a different labour. If having your first baby was difficult, of course it's harder to stay in the present and eradicate old memories. When

7

labour starts it might remind you of the first time and all the feelings that went with it. So you'll have to use all your powers of concentration. Don't anticipate during this labour—stay in the now and deal with each contraction as it comes!'

It was difficult to see how those memories could be wiped out. We thought about fear and talking about it made it seem less. Sitting in that cool room in Chelsea, where the space seemed more than it was, clasping my womb-child to stop him from further bruising my black and blue ribs, I discovered how easy it was to banish fear by bringing it into the open.

'When I was having Pete,' I told Sara, 'I completely believed I would die. Everything awful I'd ever heard about childbirth seemed to be coming true. I didn't think my body could stand it. I thought I was being ripped open and that was the only way I'd be allowed to give birth to a new life—by sacrificing my own.'

Now I think that in understanding birth it may be possible to come to terms with death. Birth and death are closely, inevitably linked in the cycles of nature. As one dies, another is born, as one is born, another dies, as one story ends, another begins. We have prolonged access to the experience of birth in a way that is denied us in death. But experiencing birth closely may help us to deal with death, since each is a confrontation with the unknown, a brush with infinity. If we want to, we can see, touch and feel birth, and then take that learning away with us to help deal with life. Its assimilation into daily living as a negative or frightening experience will have negative effects. A positive experience has positive effects.

I found that in talking to Sara about Pete's birth I could suddenly remember every detail, although until then I had buried it. Since his birth I had wanted to have children. I thought, or perhaps felt, I *should* have children, but had suffered three miscarriages. I use the word suffer because I did suffer. Not only did miscarrying hurt, but I blamed myself, because who else was there to blame? In retrospect it seems quite possible to me that repressing the terror and pain of giving birth that first time could have been in some way responsible for avoiding its recurrence. Unconsciously, I may have rejected life from my own body before it was developed enough to repeat an experience that had been so traumatic I was still in shock. I discovered with Sara that honesty and clarity are the opposites of mystification and absolutely necessary to conscious birth. It was essential to remember, and face those memories, to get rid of them.

I had found the birth of my first son painful, exhausting, frightening and lonely, because I knew absolutely nothing about what was going on inside or outside my body, what I should be doing about it or what I could expect from labour. Consequently I was shaken to the core.

The day the baby was due I was despatched to hospital by my doctor, although I had no signs of contractions. My blood pressure was up a little and I was told it would be more convenient for the doctor if I were to agree to an induction the following morning. Not knowing the pros and cons, I could not weigh them.

Labour was induced at eight in the morning. While I was under general anaesthetic, the membrane holding my waters was broken. I drowsily awoke from the drug half an hour later to find my body in the grip of something like a wrenching tool. This feeling faded, only to return in less time than I'd had to think. I realized I must be in labour, but was gasping at the violence and speed with which induction brings on contractions. I asked the nurse to call my husband and my mother, but she gave me pills instead, and my husband and mother were only allowed to stay for an hour before being sent home.

I was in labour fourteen hours under the kind of medication which made me too woolly to deal with myself or anything that was going on. Too weak to stand up for my own rights. I'd forgotten I had any rights. I didn't care how my baby was born. I was put on an intravenous drip to speed up contractions and left alone for most of the labour; shovelled from bed to stretcher to delivery table at the most intense point of discomfort, had a gas mask slapped on my face, although I summoned all remaining strength to push it away, and was oblivious when my baby was born. I felt afterwards that I had lost the whole experience. A forceps delivery bruised his minute head, scissors cut into my vagina, but he was strong and healthy and, to my dazed but infatuated eyes, perfectly beautiful. For reasons never explained to me, I was not permitted to hold my son until hours later, when he was wheeled in to me bathed and cleanly wrapped in his first trappings of so-called civilization. I had to unwrap him like a sterile parcel before I could touch his newborn skin.

I hated my husband for leaving me alone and I hated the hospital for making him go. It was incoherent hate. We had not even considered it a problem before I went into labour, simply taken it for granted that he would be there. When the hospital told him it was against its rules, he left. And I was alone. It is far from an unique story, but I am sure it brings unique pain whenever it happens. And who can tell what repercussions? The memory of pain is elusive, but the memory of desertion is sharp, and lingers. Mine are vivid memories of feeling utterly alone, of sweaty palms, clenched jaw, and the apparently impassive faces of nurses as they bent over me, uniforms crackling. 'It'll be some time yet, dear. Be a brave girl until the doctor comes. No, I don't know when he's coming. It'll be a while yet. You aren't very far along. He's a very busy man, dear.'

He had induced my baby, surely he could be there now? I got to the point when I thought I might just jump right out of the window. If only I could move. Oh God, not another one. But yes. Another one and another, and another and another till I thought I'd die if there was another, would *rather* die than stretch my body to further impossible limits.

'I wouldn't scream,' I told Sara. And she, quite rightly, put that down to my stiff-upper-lip English upbringing.

'If you don't let go, you make things worse,' she said. 'Your own noises are nothing to be afraid of.' And she'd make me grunt and groan and wail out loud, just to get used to the idea of letting rip.

'Are you afraid to make a noise when you're making love?' she asked. 'It's all part of the same principle. If you hold back, you defeat your purpose, whether it's in labour or making love. You can't flow with the natural rhythm.'

We laughed then, and I started learning how to conquer my inhibitions. It was important to be able to do it there in her living-room, not just in the privacy of my own bed, because I would have to feel free in a labour ward too.

'For a long time after Pete was born, I didn't want to make love,' I admitted. 'I didn't want to be touched. My sexuality felt bruised and I became afraid of sex in the same way I used to be as a child.'

It was a difficult admission to make. It makes me think back to that fear of surrender. I wonder if it is in all of us, the fear of letting go, of losing ourselves? Is there perhaps a link between inability to reach orgasm and inability to handle birth? Birth, orgasm, rapture, ecstasy are the rare moments when self-consciousness is lost to the winds and involuntary action takes over. Fear of one is like fear of the other. It is that sense of being overwhelmed, in space, hurtling through a time barrier—you can only go through it if you are not frightened. If you let go. And then you experience exhilaration, completion, fulfilment. It is tenseness, the terror of *not* being in control, the drawing back, which accentuates pain and sidetracks the moment of fulfilment—the ultimate orgasm—birth—the exploding galaxy of blood, membranes and *life*. Are we afraid of our natural force? Afraid of the fusion of man and woman and everything that it can mean? If we are, and we know we are, then we should try to do something to change that state. Fear of letting go is a deadly reticence which precludes total involvement and the pure experience of pleasure. In orgasm as in birth, a conscious decision leads to momentous unconscious release and feeling. The split second of joining another being in making love can be a fleeting vision which mirrors the future union of mother and child, and the separation which is also to come.

On a more practical level birth, quite as much as sex, is a genital experience. Accepting the feelings of the vaginal area has to start before we have children or we will never be able to accept the feelings of giving birth. One of the vital things which Sara taught me was how to be aware of my internal muscles, how I could tighten and relax them, how this would help me in making love and help me in giving birth.

Sara and I joined forces at a point when her strength was cool and knowing, and mine was turning a little shivery with half-remembered fear, a little sour with resentment at lack of mobility and the freedom to move at whim. There is a particular dilemma that occurs when you have known freedom and independence and then, like a bird, your wings are clipped. My first child was born before I knew or cared about establishing real individual freedom. I was one of those who thought the best I could do as a woman was to be a faithful wife and bear children. It wasn't until Peter was old enough to go to school and I had more time to myself that I found the confidence to work at something I enjoyed, journalism. When I did, it gave me a sense of my own ability, not only to create, but to survive, if necessary, alone. Although there was a child dependent on me, I did not

11

need to be dependent on anyone else. Becoming pregnant again after three miscarriages, and realizing I would carry this child full term forced a re-evaluation of my own immediate reality.

Society is far less able to accept working independence in a woman pregnant than in one who is not. The fact may not hit you until you show that you have conceived. Realization of the limits imposed by pregnancy dawns when your stomach swells to a size that hampers physical movement, so provoking uncomfortable reaction in the people around you. Until then, the dream of new life blooming inside you has the unreal quality of something intensely private, unseen and maybe only slightly felt.

Perhaps it is more difficult to deal with being pregnant if you have already fought to establish independence from role-playing, than it is if your existence has always been geared entirely to motherhood. I know that the larger I became with Orion, the more cumbersome I felt, the less free. Before I met Sara, and could talk about it, I was beginning to feel both vulnerable and dependent, although I recognized they were the very conditions I had spent years trying to escape. Being with another woman who understood what I was going through made it easier to confront myself. One day I had to sit down and take a good look at the fact that not only was I pregnant, but I was going to go through labour, and I was going to have this child. That would mean big changes in my ideas of freedom, my desire to work, my ability to give. Having learned how to fight to be myself, I was going to have to learn how to accept, in order to be myself. It was an interesting challenge, and in exploring it, I came closer to understanding my female receptive nature.

Acceptance is not the same as passivity, but we confuse them sometimes, and perhaps that is why women of action cannot reconcile themselves easily to a condition that requires them to be still and take stock of who they are and what they are doing. Accepting that a woman is biologically fashioned to receive rather than penetrate does not mean giving up all claim to independence. Having been penetrated and planted with seed, we do not then lose our creative energies, we have to rechannel them. Pregnant, I have to accept that I received that male sperm because it was my choice to be there on that bed that floor that field that mountain top under that torrent of tumbling water that crescent moon that blazing sunset in that sweaty turmoil that tender cushion of roses with that man at that time and something within me *came to life* because of the deliberate act of receiving.

Sometimes it is hard to take that acceptance is important to peace of mind, and the relentless way birth edges closer in the last months of pregnancy can freeze you into impotent resentment if you do not see what is happening and learn the value of acceptance in alleviating stress.

Like many others I felt I had lost touch with myself through carrying another being. That my hold on known reality was tenuous. I would waver from glory as my tits swelled and my skin glowed, to despair as my moods rocketed this way and that, my nails cracked, hair fell out, teeth chipped and clumsiness doubled. Half the time, I stubbornly refused to behave as though anything had happened to change my status or size. Quarter of the time, I collapsed in a pathetic heap of self-pity. Quarter of the time, I was helpless with laughter. Sara pointed out that the ratio was all wrong. I should be laughing more.

Humour gave me a new slant on pregnancy. I began to take it all less seriously. The child lay less heavy on my stomach, responsibility lighter on my shoulders, fear was flushed out of memory with the hope of being able to change the pattern this time. And through constant practice, both with Sara and at home, the 'conscious controlled' breathing eventually became second nature.

It was reassuring to be reminded that my condition was not isolated unless I insisted on making it so. Other women were going through the same changes, being put to the same tests, being given the same gifts. I was learning that having a baby could mean having a good time. Companionship made this possible. Sara helped my life become a preparation for birth, first when I was pregnant with Orion, and then later when I was pregnant with Liam. She taught me how to relax and laugh and spill out my hopes and dreams. We shook out a few skeletons in both our cupboards. I found that one of the greatest joys when you are pregnant is sharing the things you go through with someone who knows what you are talking about.

In those last few weeks of carrying Orion, when my breath was short and my belly like a globe, I learned how the state of my mind influenced the state of my body and how the two are inescapably connected. I understood that my own insecurities might be intensified many times in the womblife of my child, and gained a necessary

13

perspective when the waves of self-pity peculiar to pregnancy threatened to swamp my equilibrium. Other people are like mirrors, and we need to see our reflection.

Sara and I met as friends and learned from each other. We wrangled and tested and probed and exchanged, so the time spent together was stimulating and fun. The last slow weeks of heaviness passed in a flash of friendship as we moved to a common goal. She talked to me almost as much as I talked to her and because I learned not only from, but about her, it was always interesting, and the flow of energy between us was properly balanced. The secret was exchange, the support companionship, the key honesty, the structure flexible, the environment relaxing.

Wanting to share the preparation for birth sets up the conditions for honesty. Having a baby is not the time for playing elaborate games, with yourself or anyone else. In preparing for Orion alone with Sara, and Liam with Sara and several other people, I could never get away with throwaway remarks. Not for a minute could I say 'Christ, I'm fed up with the kids,' or 'I'm really off sex,' without Sara confronting me with the reality of the statement. 'Do you really mean that?' 'Why is it happening?' 'Does anyone else feel the same way?' It was provocative, but vital to the development of self-awareness. Her reasoning is that if you are frustrated, don't lock it in, let it out. Her challenges were often accompanied by a brisk invitation to punch out frustration on a pillow. This is a Reichian method of releasing tension that Sara learned while in therapy in California. I find it works wonders to this day. Better a pummelled pillow than a battered baby.

So the preparation taught me to know my body, ease my mind, tone my muscles, control my breathing, grasp the ebb and flow of muscles contracting separately from a whole organism, and how best to treat myself and child with care.

For the first time I began seriously considering the food I put into my system. Being so aware of the child growing inside encouraged a self-discipline I had never exercised before. I learned that the placenta, the fleshy part of your womb to which the baby is linked by the umbilical cord, is more like a sponge than a barrier. It will not protect your child from any muck you put into yourself, it absorbs it, and so does the baby. The realization brought some longstanding indulgences to an abrupt halt. I no longer had only myself to be responsible for. Although eating for two is a big mistake, nourishing for two is essential.

I avoided chemicals as much as I could—tricky in this tin-can plastic supermarket city-living age—but once you start thinking about how much healthier fresh vegetables must be than tinned, you start reading the labels on the tins, and that is enough to put anyone off. Alcohol made me throw up immediately, so that was easy to cross off the list. The faintest whiff of nicotine made me push away smouldering cigarette butts and rush to the rubbish bin with half-empty ashtrays. Heartburn and constipation were two of the most undignified blights of my pregnancies, so, despite cravings for jacket potatoes, I levelled out my diet to a fairly even balance, and quickly began to sense what I really needed.

I felt the baby strong inside me and he gave me strength. The nest into which I was to bring him was growing shakier and shakier, as the distance between his father and myself grew wider. I wept sometimes and shook the kaleidoscope of my mind to see which way the pieces would fall and which way the picture made more sense. There was never a straight answer. The imponderables led me a fancy dance. And although I felt very much alone at the beginning, there was always this compulsion to have the child. It was as though he had made up his own mind from the very beginning and was simply waiting for me to accept the wisdom of intuition.

Doctors had told me I would have difficulty carrying a baby full term, having had three miscarriages, with a gap of eight years between the birth of this child and the last. I was advised to stay in bed for most of the pregnancy and have an operation to stitch the neck of the uterus, which might not be strong enough to hold the growing baby. But I felt that to put in the stitch would be to interfere, perhaps too much, in the careful work of the womb. It was possible the operation might *cause* a miscarriage. It was also possible that staying in bed for nine months would mean my muscles were not adequately rehearsed for labour's heavy duty. So even at the onset of pregnancy I was torn many ways, and in the end decided the only thing to do was to follow my instincts and see where nature took the pregnancy. Medical guidance had not prevented the three previous miscarriages. It seemed there was no way of knowing who knew more about my body—me or the doctors. I decided to back myself.

This was the point at which I realized the power of intuition, inner tuition, and that at a certain stage in the making of difficult decisions, you have to balance the inner voice with the outer ones that cannot know you as well as you do. Much to the astonishment of my doctor, I went into hospital when I was over three months pregnant, having allowed myself to be talked into doing something I didn't really want to do, and then left again the same night, before having the stitch operation. I was suddenly convinced in the metallic clang of the ward that I did not have the right to subject my unborn child to the interference of an instrument that could cause damage—if leaving it to nature would not, in itself, be mortally dangerous. However carefully the instrument was inserted, there was a danger that it might either displace the life already growing there, or imprison one which was not forming properly and nature would eventually reject. My doctor explained each aspect of the situation quite clearly when I finally demanded it—and allowed me to make my own decision when I also finally demanded that right. It is not a decision, or a realization, I have ever regretted.

From then on I lived my pregnant life as naturally as possible. I took care of my health, without being fussy. I avoided the obvious provocations of miscarriage such as drugs, alcohol, violent sex, riding horses, long journeys in rackety cars or bumpy bicycle rides. But I ran up and down stairs, walked for miles, danced through the nights, climbed the highest mountain on Ibiza at full moon, and was healthier than I had been for years. By the time I met Sara, I knew I was going to make it this time and was both nervous and glad.

At the day of his birth I was strong and fit and knew how to control my breathing. Through growing awareness of my female nature, I gained a confidence which gave me strength. Much earlier in the pregnancy, the man who was then my husband, Michael, and I had decided to separate in all but the sharing of a roof. Now I was able to persuade him to join me for the birth of his child. I was falling in love with John, an American I met early in my pregnancy, after my marriage had begun to fall apart. Now I encouraged both him and Michael to share the birth of this baby, who *belonged* to no one, but was being given life through me. Feeling so much love in myself, towards the baby and the two men closest to us, Orion and I received, in that last month of his gestation, a kind of comfort without commitment that I had never expected, but really enjoyed. The men rallied in the excitement of the approaching birth, so that when the time came for me to go into labour it seemed simple to us that we all share in the celebration of a new life.

All three of us went to the hospital, and amazingly the staff did not turn either man away. Sara came too. As a friend. We had been through so much already. I wanted her support to complete the cycle. My doctor was ready. The hospital knew I had been taking lessons in breathing and natural birth with Sara, and I had explained very carefully beforehand that I would want the father of my child to be present. The doctor didn't know about John, but he didn't even raise an eyebrow. I suppose he was used to my peculiarities, having seen me go in and out of hospital in one night when he thought he was to perform an operation on me.

I told the astonished faces of the nurses that Sara was my teacher, essential for the natural birth of the child, that John was my astrologer, essential for the charting of his horoscope, and that Michael was the father, essential for a loving birth. We took it blithely for granted that there could be no objections. Riding high on the gust of energy that I'd sucked in from heaven to blow out my baby, we sailed along corridors carrying pillows and incense, pausing only for me to breathe through a contraction.

When our coterie arrived on the labour floor and stated its business, the old black midwife laughed and loved it all, saying it was natural I should want to have my baby natural. Two of the younger nurses looked prim, but no aura of disapproval could stop the cavalcade. Which shows that almost all you need to break down barriers is the wish to do so and a flair for street theatre. People *like* to be surprised by happiness.

If you are nervous of hospitals and all that starch and uniformity and routine, forget it. You know you. *You* are having the baby. Don't let them make you just another little bolt in their great big tidy hospital clickity-clack machine. You are at the apex of alchemical force. Within your body another body has begun to move out to fulfil its destiny on earth. Get on with the miracle. Miracles break all the rules.

Conscious birth taught me that secret. Seven months pregnant, I was like a bird in captivity, beating my wings against a cage of frustration. By the eighth I was flying away. My baby was born in the

17

full floodlight of the moon. I named him after a constellation and caught a glimpse of why we are here.

* * *

Barely a year after Orion's birth I was pregnant again. It wasn't planned. I became pregnant despite the coil. Ninety-eight per cent of the time it is safe, they tell me. A two per cent chance, yet my third son, Liam, came determinedly into the world on the 8th August, 1972. My smiling little sunshine Leo who came out blinking bright, not crying, more totally aware of aeons past and diamond present than anyone I have ever felt. Light of my life, whose father held his head as he spurted out of me into the harshness of neonworld. My only regret is that we could not have been at home, that he could not have been welcomed by soft lights and roses as he lay on my breast, the two of us held together by our life cord still, he looking me clear in the eye, going back in blue timelessness to knowledge I may never see again.

Afterwards they took him from me. Cut the cord and placed his frail five pounds in a glass box instead of letting me hold him close with my warmth. His mouth turned to find my nipple and sucked only air. Seeing this, I later broke the rules, and crept to the glass box which separated us. I asked the nurse to let me hold him. He took the nourishment which had waited so long and they didn't take him away from me again. This third baby had both his parents present from beginning to end, conception to birth. Our own union consolidated by sharing so completely the making of a child. John came with me to classes, held my hand through the sickness, brewed special teas, kept alcohol away, watched my diet by doing the shopping, remembered the vitamins for me, washed my hair, oiled my skin, paced my breathing, touched gently the swell in my stomach as it moved in the night, and loved me tender through it all.

There were medical complications. My ankles and fingers puffed up and I knew something was wrong when I had to have my favourite silver ring cut off. There is a difference between feet swelling in summer heat, and feet swelling in pregnancy, for this can be one of the signs of the condition known as toxemia. The hospital checked and said I should rest, for I might be at risk. Toxemia is a serious disturbance of the body's metabolism which, if allowed to develop, can among other things affect the circulation of the blood to the baby. In its most extreme form it can lead to death of both mother and child. The crucial thing is to delay its development. If you know what to look out for, this is easy to do with good medical advice and common sense. I do not think English hospitals really explain this hazard to women either strongly enough or early enough in pregnancy. I am making a strong point of it now because I was told that I had high blood pressure and might be at risk from toxemia, but no one ever explained what that meant. I had no idea it could be really dangerous, until after Liam was born. Perhaps if I had been aware of it sooner, I might have paid more attention to resting.

In fact, when I was eight months pregnant, I went for a check-up just before moving to the country with the rest of my family to spend the waiting weeks away from the city scrum, and was told that I would have to go into hospital immediately. My blood pressure was too high and there was albumin in my urine. The doctor informed me that I would stay there for a few days, and if my blood pressure did not go down, I would have an induction.

Now, as happens with so many women I have known, there was some confusion about the dates, no one was quite sure when the baby was due, and I hated the idea of my baby's life journey being started artificially. Reluctantly I went into hospital, knowing I had less chance of warding off induction once I was inside.

On the first night I went to sleep wondering if I would be there for weeks until he was born. If hospital rest was the only way to avoid induction, then I was prepared to wait it out. About midnight I woke with a peculiarly familiar feeling. I couldn't get to sleep again, and by two in the morning I knew the baby was coming of its own accord. It took several more hours to convince the duty nurse that I was having slight contractions. Only after examining me internally would she accept that I was right. Then the doctor thought it was much too soon to have the baby. In his judgement the child would be so premature it would need an incubator and intensive care unit, so he wanted to give me sedatives in the hope that contractions would cease.

It is hard to explain to anyone that you know inside you that your child is ready to be born. But I knew. The certainty stopped me from panicking with the doctors, allowed me to relax through the gentle contractions that continued all day without bothering me. By the late afternoon they were quite strong and coming quite quickly. This time I had to convince the doctors that in less than a few hours I was actually going to have a baby. When they eventually wheeled me into the delivery room I was overtaken by extreme chills and started shaking like a leaf. Apparently it is a common emotional reaction in childbirth, possibly linked to toxemia, and not really serious, only no one got round to explaining that to me until after the baby was born. If I had not known how to relax into the shivering, it would have been very difficult to cope; but as it was, the breathing took me through all the changes with an equanimity I had hardly known I possessed.

The fears that held me back from enjoying the first birth, eased by the second and disappeared by the third. Sara was not there to guide me with Liam, but John was, and much stronger this time, it being his baby and there being no one but he and I and our child locked in the life struggle. The movements and energy of birth flowed freely through my body so that the child came smoothly into the world, swifter than I'd dreamed possible, with so little pain that its memory is like the brush of a feather across my skin.

He was small, but not too small, and astoundingly healthy.

I found the awareness of life that came with being conscious for the births of my two youngest sons was like turning a key in the centre of myself, so that suddenly, click, I became whole and understood the meaning of being a mother. It is not bondage, but a natural part of me, a woman, that was missing before and now takes me nearer completion. In learning the positive side of having babies I have grown closer to all my children and my man.

Most of my life I had thought I wasn't maternal. Children, babies, didn't turn me on. I briefly glanced at the total involvement some women had with theirs, the joy it seemed to bring them, and the frustration seeping out of others. It didn't seem to touch me either way. The glance was cursory and detached. There was no desire to explore it further until the blurred confusion of Peter's birth eventually prepared me for holding Orion in my arms, having watched him come out of me.

It was not that I did not love my first child in his early years, rather that I didn't know what to do with him, didn't know how to relate to him as closely as I wanted to, and didn't discover how simple it is until I had experienced birth fully, on every level, suppressing and repressing nothing. Since then, the cold distance between me and babies has melted. I do not think there is such a being as the ideal mother, although some women obviously have stronger maternal instincts than others. I know I am often impatient with my brood. But never cold again. Never unmoved.

One of the first things I noticed about Sara was her friendship with her children, not suffocating smother-love, but companionship that left room for freak-outs and was based on honesty. She enjoyed her children without letting them hang onto her apron strings and frazzle her edges. An independent hen with independent chicks, yet the family ties were stronger than most I had come across—and invisible. It gave me hope for my future role as mother of more than one.

No one can tell you how it is to be a mother, or a father for that matter. I can only point out that it hasn't tied me down. Likewise, I cannot explain the experience of giving birth; simply tell how it was for me and give you some guidelines and information I think will help. In the end, personal experience is the only kind of knowledge one can absolutely believe in. The rest is conjecture, memories, dreams and visions.

We can help each other just by being together—a man and a woman—a woman and a woman—two couples—three or four couples—a pregnant woman and a sister with children—mother and daughter . . . the combinations are infinite. It helps to share, to be loving, to exchange ideas, barter clothes, compare experience, provoke thought, practise skills with other people so you don't take the easy way out and regret it later. I found that if people get together to go through a preparation like this, they can laugh away some of the fear inbred in us. The currents of contact are kept alive by interaction between individuals who really believe there are things to be done that can humanize the course and conditions of childbirth in this mechanized age.

Experience is more fun than theorizing, and more enlightening. Awareness is an education in itself. Action is reality. Like Lao-tzu: 'The way to do is to be.' I learned that to participate in birth I must be prepared.

But this preparation, and the illuminating experience it led to, has taken me further. I question the increasingly technological routine of modern birth. Natural childbirth has been an ideal for several decades, achieved by few in the Western world and now rapidly being eroded. New drugs, new machines, bigger more centralized institutions are designed to reduce mortality, but in fact they now threaten to swamp the family. So to achieve Naturebirth today, we must raise the question of the rights of men and women to bear children as they wish. We must challenge the status quo in childbirth, weigh the benefits of mechanization and discover ways to rehumanize birth. Once convinced of the ideal, we must find practical ways of making it a reality. A preparation based on the integration of mind and body by learning awareness of the deeper mysteries of both can lead us to Naturebirth.

I
Naturebirth
A Necessary Ideal

1

Birth Rights

I want to broaden the concept of women's liberation so that women who are mothers do not feel excluded by the forthright singleness of those who normally carry its banner.

I think female emancipation has to go further and mean more than political, sexual or financial freedom. It has to embrace motherhood, which means we must reinterpret the role of mother so that those who see families as traps can see the ways to enjoy having children. This new freedom has to come from female understanding of the female psyche and anatomy, because self-awareness does not split the two. So that woman in her most womanly of states, pregnant, can choose independence at the height of dependence, mobility in physical restriction, sexuality with serenity, wholeness despite invasion, privacy in unsevered companionship, oneness in duality, escape from the unavoidable, change in the seemingly immutable.

In half a century, women have pushed themselves from the railings of Downing Street right into the Houses of Parliament; from the green lawns of suburbia into the Capitol. They have pushed their earnings up and their limits down; they have infiltrated, against great opposition, industry, the professions and the arts. Those women who have been strong enough to campaign against the odds for a cause that will take years to manifest itself on a universal level have helped make it possible for others to have more choice in their life than ever before.

We have choice through birth control, we have choice through the legislation on abortion, we have the choice of our mates because marriages are no longer arranged nor escorts vetted, and living with someone outside marriage no longer means complete social ostracization.

Emancipation may come when we are not simply young and free and beautiful in our rebellion. Perhaps it comes when we are not single, not free from commitment, but still strong; when we are mothers who do not see in that state something lost but something gained.

Germaine Greer, sister-at-arms to Women's Liberation, wrote that she thought women would consider marriage and motherhood less of a duty, a yoke and a trap, if they knew more about how to enjoy it. I am sure that is true. But her concept of liberated motherhood is escape to fantasy. Her idea of the family is the freedom to run from it. Her ideal runs to communes: in idyllic sunplaces children run naked amid lemon trees; no one mother has more or less responsibility for any child, no one child has call on his or her blood parents above the rest of the community, so that precious mobility is bought at the price of eternal love. I don't believe in that because I have children and I don't want it. Some might. *My* conviction is that our children are not our bondage but our hope, and birth is where it all begins.

Time has taught me to be wary of extremes and causes. On the rebound from violent affairs with radical thought, minds so often snap further back than before. Kicking over establishments leaves huge holes for new ones. Human nature changes very slowly when human needs do not vary much; lately our needs have altered as fast as our culture. Awareness of these needs is evolution. Action through awareness is what brings change; revolution, *revolving*, speaks of wheels, turns in time and comes back, spiralling, to another place.

The late 1960s saw a social revolution. Middle-class youth moved away from the impositions of its heritage. Out of their disillusion came the voice of the peaceful alternative. Suddenly there were liberation movements, a growing newly articulated dissatisfaction with politics, politicians and policies. It became urgently necessary to reform Civil Rights and there was noisy protest against the war in Vietnam, the space programme, racial discrimination, Presidents, Popes and Prime Ministers.

It was a psycho-sexual revolution fed by the common and shattering experience of altering consciousness, often by means of mind-expanding drugs. Most of those who turned on to grass and were an active part of the Sixties realized that they had forgotten how simple life is. Raising consciousness was an effort to keep in touch with that knowledge. Trekking back to nature through walls of plastic, the psychedelic experience gave a glimpse of how life could be, and united those who had seen that vision more strongly than those who had not seen it had bargained for. Dogged by the spiritual poverty of Western capitalism, thousands upon thousands of young people dropped out of a system they had been bred to believe would bind them forever. They side-stepped a world where no one seemed to laugh very much, and moved to country places and sun islands and alien cultures where the pace was slower, the air less polluted, the food organic, the demands more logical and there seemed to be time to enjoy what was left of the planet.

It was escape from unpleasant reality; but life didn't stay simple long. People found that they really could not live with *no* money, since they had not managed to loosen the stranglehold of the stock markets. They could not survive if they gave *everything* away, because there was always someone who took a bit too much, who did not return in kind, who could not contribute enough. You had to have a passport to travel. You do get busted if you break the law. Bureaucracy can always reduce you to a number. Somehow. You still have to have food inside you and clothes to keep you warm, and while you could grow food in the country, or make clothes, you still needed raw materials, so you still had to work for someone who had money, so you were back in the system you despised. The alternative to that was guns. Some people crossed the hairline barrier between the dream of revolution and the violent deed, and many died martyrs for a cause they could barely formulate.

One set of values raucously put down—another set eagerly clung to. Dope and free speech, a change in the laws concerning obscenity, homosexuality, abortion and divorce. Nixon withdrew troops from Vietnam and the American people withdrew from Nixon. Power to the people, but the people had to live.

So an alternative system was devised, though few realized it was a system. Shaped by the hippy intelligentsia—those of the movement intelligent and willing enough to articulate its aims—and who did little but that. And given substance by the hippy bourgeoisie. They, like their reviled forebears, had money. Because they didn't like living without it. Theirs is a creative culture out of which has come music, which makes money; and newspapers, which make money;

27

and drug-dealing, which makes money. There are now alternative lawyers to defend the lawbreakers, doctors to treat and supply them, a political system which can ignore them because they want to be ignored and can afford to pay for it.

And so too the women's movements of today, bringing their own revolution, in women's rights, run the risk of setting up such extreme roles that the 'liberated' woman becomes another stereotype. History has pulverized woman's psychic powers and offered up femininity impaled on a stake and labelled witch; has forced us into the kitchen when we wanted the bedroom, and brought us to bed with child when we wanted man. Women's liberation proclaims an end to that. But the missing spark from women's liberation seems to be understanding of the receptive element in women's nature; and it is woman's appreciation of this which could transform drudgery into positive action.

So when I think about change, I will not turn my back too finally on past ideas of how it should feel to be woman and mother, lest I find I've pivoted right round on my heel, and am building again the structures that bound me. I'll try to learn from the old and the new, and adapt.

Giving birth has the inherent duality of being at once unique to each woman and universal to all women. The experience divides and unites us. I think it would divide us less, were more women to understand that its simple yet intricate natural process can give a new dimension to the quality of life. I have seen childbirth mark the transition of girl to woman. If the transition is to be complete, the creative aspect of the receptive function must be understood. In accepting receptivity, we become creative.

This does not mean that I believe woman's only contribution and salvation is bearing children. If I did, I wouldn't be writing this book in between scribbling articles, researching figures, cooking meals, looking at schools, attending seminars, feeding babies, making love, studying music, getting into arguments, flying a plane and giving preparation classes. But I do believe that, once chosen, pregnancy, motherhood, having babies, can and should be a significant learning experience. It can teach you about yourself, your relation to your body, your man, your mother, your children, your family, the world. It is an experience the creative moment of which does not finish at birth, but is endless.

To me, real liberation is understanding the right of choice. Liberated women with an identity of their own have usually chosen to bear a child. For every woman it means adjustment and reassessment. The single state is radically different from that of the vessel which nourishes another life. Pregnancy is time to acknowledge that we can not only enjoy our female essence single, but also united, doubled, with seed inside ripening and bursting into new form; and see also how we must protect that seed.

So, new age woman, with your pen and rifle, needle and cheque book, car and coil, wiles and intellect, your politics and passion, your bisexuality and high sensuality and sharp sensibility, your cunningly juggled male/female identity, your constant attempt to balance the creative and receptive, and your search for freedom through wisdom, the time has come to *like* being a woman, and all that entails. To enjoy being a mother, not resent it, enjoy giving birth, not reject it.

It doesn't make sense to be a street revolutionary crying out for awareness, if you are not aware when your children are born. It doesn't help evolution to fight chemical poisoning and try to preserve land resources, if we cannot recognize and deal with the pollution of birth dehumanized by machine. The overriding dangers are the same: we will become secondary to the machines we make.

Although medicine has achieved great scientific breakthroughs for humanity, the prevailing attitude of most modern obstetrics towards the birth of our children is less than humanitarian. It is often not only insensitive to the needs of woman and child, but perilously narrow-minded, so stuck in established routine that a change in viewpoint cannot be countenanced.

Acknowledging that progress in civilization has not necessarily meant progress for the unborn and newly born child will help parents understand the complexity which faces them in bearing children today. Today's culture presents them with a subtle and complicated set of problems, because our whole lives are more complicated than they have ever been. We no longer tell the time by the sun and chart our course by the stars, we build intricate mechanisms to do those jobs, mechanisms that need careful handling, and can go wrong. The same goes for the way we light our houses. Living as I do for part of the year on an island where we have no electricity, I know that candles are easier to deal with than wires that short, plugs that fuse—and huge bills from the Electricity Board. And so also with babies. If you are a normally healthy woman, concerned with keeping yourself normally healthy while you carry a child, it is much simpler to have your baby naturally if you can, than to be dependent on men *and* machines. What retrogression that is, for women to surrender to man-handled devices and drugs. With the introduction of machinery into birth there is very little information for either women or doctors to refer back to, no historical pattern with which to compare notes, indeed little long-term research. Yet think what is at stake: the well-being of your child. Nature has been tested. We know what works and, of course, what doesn't. Birth technology has not had that time. Where we can rely on nature, we should.

The mechanization of birth has come about very quickly. Machines have crept up on us almost before we knew it. Some of the devices used now look like space fiction compared to the relatively mundane weirdness of the machinery I encountered in my own first labour—so we are talking about a period of roughly a decade. Techniques and attitudes seem to have acquired a progressively more steely impersonality and dedication to regime, which has encouraged women to relinquish individuality and block feeling. I think it's very dangerous, and I don't mind being emotional about it. My child, my feelings, my life and the health of my family are at stake. I see drugs and mechanical devices developed for helping the sick and diagnosing disease being used with alarmingly little discrimination between normal and abnormal pregnancy. Few doctors bother to explain their effect on women or their babies, so parents have to demand that information, to realize it is their right to know and that it is necessary. If the facts of modern birth are hidden, there is no basis for men and women to make a true decision as to how they have their children.

A woman should have the right to choose the conditions in which she gives birth, and a right to the information relevant to making that choice. It could make the difference between birth being a constricting or a liberating experience, one that is healthy or damaging for herself and the child, one for which she is aware or unaware. A woman prepared and wanting conscious birth must have the right to insist on recognition of her innate natural knowledge of herself and her child. Mechanized culture has led to mechanized birth, but nature cannot be totally replaced by machinery.

I believe we can improve the conditions of pregnancy and birth by closer contact with the process of nature in carrying and bringing forth life. We should be able to marry old knowledge with new discoveries; technology with nature. It is a fallacy to assume that technology is always synonymous with efficiency, sometimes it is, but sometimes it is not. If nature and technology were harnessed more often than pitted against one another, as is the custom, then it should be possible to manifest this marriage of science with intuition in a practical way. Through my own experience and experiment, and the work and research of other women, of psychiatrists, paediatricians and a few enlightened obstetricians concerned with finding a balance between these forces, I have come to the conclusion that childbirth sets the mould for future living and may well affect the foundations of the family. So the need to find balance at the beginning of life is urgent. In looking for the magic formula, this combination of man-made miracles and the unarguable inexplicable miracle of nature, we have to explore both. In doing this one sees that it is foolish, even dangerous, to abuse or dismiss either.

New technology has blunted our awareness of ourselves and the primitive functions of our lives. The rites of birth, copulation and death have lost some sensibility to the march of science. We have allowed our animal instincts to be subdued. They are not 'nice'. Feeling, but not understanding, their loss, we resort to artificial provocation, titillation, hoping somewhere to evoke forgotten spirit and passion. See it in the polluted river of pornography and narcotics, see people watching the endless bloody sagas of war, numbed by their atrocities. The escape then is to superficiality, automation, plastic make-believe.

If we plasticize our dead—and the cosmetic burial grounds of Forest Lawn, where corpses are ornately raped before interment, have waiting-lists of undead thousands, wishing last wishes for the macabre rearrangement of time's life sentence—then what are we doing to our newly born? Plastic corpses, plastic babies. If any more pharmaceutical substances and any more machines dictate the course of any more births, when it is beyond the realm of computer-duty, then we must face the implications of tampering with nature.

The solution to the imbalance between nature and birth technology that we have now lies in educating women both to have confidence

31

in their own instinct and their ability to bring forth life, and to reach for full information about the medical processes to which they are exposed or to which they might have to resort. A vital part of such education is the awareness that psychic and physical feelings are inseparable, the conscious and the subconscious interact constantly. A woman who knows her mind can manage her body. The value of being prepared for birth is that a woman who understands what is happening to her and why, what she wants to put into and take out of the experience, is better equipped to deal with the unknown element, than a woman who is not conscious of such things.

Women functioning in this state of heightened consciousness while giving birth are also more likely to realize the relative roles of male and female during birth, and probably more able to turn on the men who father their children and the physicians who attend them, to their rights to have a baby when, where, how and with whom they wish. Hopefully members of the medical profession will listen to this statement, but I'm convinced it is only parents of the new generations who will turn this from dream to reality. Once women know what they need, they can alert both doctors and fathers to those needs, so that with them they may decree and alter the conditions of birth.

Female power has been denigrated so long, been so shrouded in secrecy and suspicion that to an astonishing number of men it is still a threat, and the intimate ritual of birth not something to be shared but feared, an unseeable female act performed behind closed doors out of sight and sound. Yet all the fathers I know who are present at the birth of their children seem to have a deeper connection with both mother and child than the man who waits outside. The traditional figure of the father who still paces the corridors with bitten nails while mother struggles heroically behind those closed doors, is like an out-of-date comic strip, born of chauvinism and perpetuated by habit, the all-too-human habit of following a system. We can kick the habit and change the system. If we want to. Although as a race we are nurtured on medicine that in practice concentrates more on blanking out symptoms than uprooting causes and although childbirth is still apparently all too often treated by mothers-to-be and medical profession alike as an affliction, with women as patients rather than mothers, there are alternatives to the cold and scary mechanics of modern birth, and it is up to us to find them.

If a man makes sure he is with his woman when their child is born, and a woman makes sure that come hell or highwater no job, no friend, no enemy, no outside force or institutional rule will keep a father away from his child at birth, then the part a man plays has myriad reflections in time. He is mate and friend, guide and nurse, father and lover, voice and echo and hopefully continues to be. Most important, in labour, he is translator. If he shares the preparation, he will know what you know, why you know it, why he knows it, and what you both are and want. It puts him in the position of being the most accurate mediator between mother and doctor. The father of the newborn is as essential to its present and future life as the mother. Whenever possible, his energy should be part of the baby's welcome.

I found that sharing the birth of my two youngest children was an extraordinary celebration, the fulfilment of love. I think many people have found and will find in shared birth something they have never quite reached before. Call it what you will, logically sharing is an essential part of love and family life.

In the old days, the family was found to be the best form of social structure for people to live in, because it was easy to live and work together, bound by common goals and sharing common land and food. Now that balance of survival has been tampered with. We are in such a muddle that the nuclear family is constantly split by divorce, maimed by greed, unable to put down roots because there are so few shared moments, so little direct sensual contact. It is no longer the custom to hold your child immediately at birth. Few women breastfeed. Men seldom see their wives and children in the hustle to get out of the house and into the office—a major percentage of their time is spent away from the home. The family is remote, little wonder that birth is too.

Changing that means reversing conditioning. Almost anything men and women do can be done with children alongside. It is a question of habit. You can get used to anything and you can change habits. It is modern habit for a man to walk out of the door every morning and wave goodbye to his family, and woman's habit to get stuck with the nappies. Breaking that pattern is difficult, but not impossible.

We should try to find an alternative. If we fall in love with our children by watching their birth, why should we be content to be separated from them from then onwards if we want to continue to develop as individuals? Why should we be content to accept a job, or an academic opportunity, at the sacrifice of parenthood? Why don't universities, colleges, offices and factories provide more facilities for children, so that working need not mean breaking up the family, so that a man is free to see the birth of his child, so that a woman can keep her baby with her, whatever she is doing? We the parents have to make that a reality.

It is crucial to understand birth because it affects, literally, the future of mankind. If we are to consider that our children are influenced for the rest of their lives by the way they are born (and the experience of psychologists suggests that they can be), then as parents we have the responsibility of influencing the way they are born for the better, or neurosis will continue to go hand in hand with psychosis, suppression continue to lead to depression. Is it possible that autistic children actually choose to keep quiet, not wanting to express themselves, because feeling was stifled at birth— they were cut off, first from the mother, and through that from themselves? I believe that preparation for birth might prevent such misery and a welcoming birth could improve life.

We should think about the sensitivity of a new being moving from one element, water, to another, air, perhaps even from one dimension, outside time, to another, within our man-made measurement of time—and then think about the welcome that is customary today: the metal instruments, harsh lights, and impersonal handling of the institutionalized births our culture insists are necessary. We can change those conditions by changing our attitude to birth.

We should consider the psyche of a woman, and prepare it for feeling; understand the body of a woman, and prepare it for feeling; make contact with the senses of the unborn and the newborn; be conscious of the nature of our bodies and the awakening of our wombchildren; be prepared for the difficulties of holding onto the natural through the welter of mechanical medical devices, be prepared, man and woman, to share in the first moments of a child's life.

Psychiatrists, such as Freud, Reich, Reik and Jung have labelled birth 'trauma'—a morbid condition of the body caused by wound or external violence—an emotional shock. It may be both. It need not be either. The choice is yours. A morbid condition so embedded within us that we play it out again and again, the conditioned neurosis of the mother becoming the psychosis of the child. Or a moment of ecstasy. If we are ready for the birth of our children, we will know enough to prevent the busy thoughtlessness of strangers from interfering in the delicate arrangements of first living moments.

One doctor to make a written plea for less intervention in birth was Grantly Dick-Read. Nearly forty years ago he wrote that childbirth was one of the highest points of human spiritual achievement:

> '. . . the birth of a child is an emotional experience which brings with it all the noblest and most loving qualities of men, women and children. It unearths the fund of tenderness, companionship and understanding that smooths our social structure and brings confidence to replace suspicion . . .'

His theme was that although obstetrics took care of the physical components of reproduction, it had no comprehension of the spiritual and therefore made no allowance for it. He did much to liberate women from the exclusively male chauvinist attitudes of the medical profession then—from what men thought childbirth should be. He articulated powerful resentment of the way the wishes and aims of mothers were discounted, and began the laborious job of paving a route towards childbirth alternative to the glossy maze of exclusively scientific achievement. He suggested, even then, that it might be better for women to *feel* birth.

His message was crucial, but his was a voice in the wilderness. In many and different ways it still is today. Developments in medicine have assumed formidable scientific authority that is harder to question than ever before; the male-dominated medical profession still wields unchallenged power in childbirth; women still fail to voice their fundamental rights in this supremely female experience. And the newborn is usually bundled like an unfeeling object.

A woman who sees childbirth as potentially one of the greatest events in her life can take advantage of that which others have learned of the event. She can liberate not only her child but herself, her sensations, her expression, her energy, her strength—joined by man as partner, lover, doctor, friend, rather than dictated to by man as professional stranger.

If she understands clearly that she does have the right of choice in how she gives birth, that it is, in fact, her child's birth right, then she can extend the concept of emancipation by making a reality of Naturebirth.

2

The Status Quo In Question

Should Men Direct Birth?

I know how strange it is to be attended by masked men when you are having a baby; to be told what to do and how to do it by those who have never and will never give birth. It is one of the more peculiar and unnerving aspects of modern childbirth.

Touch is vital during birth. Senses so sensitive they could break. How many men in white coats can really feel that? They, who have never known what it is to move in labour and bring forth life? What logic is there to an unknown man presiding over an unknown catharsis, possibly shutting out the known father of the child, the mother and sisters of the woman, the females of the family who might comfort with their common wisdom?

When I was giving birth, I wanted my mother and my lover. I wanted loving familiar faces. Strangers and uniforms seemed grotesque accompaniments to the intimate rite of birth. We may be saving lives by modernizing birth procedures, but we may also be losing understanding of how life should be. It has taken a few short hectic years to destroy the tradition of centuries. Women have almost completely lost touch with each other in the only experience that men cannot have. It is too often routine now, that men are the deliverers and women the passive attendants to birthing, a regime which does little to take into account the feelings of the woman giving birth.

From the earliest days it has been the custom for women, usually the elders of the family, to gather for the ritual of birth and preside over delivery of the children. Even if they had no previous knowledge of medicine, they would have the practical knowledge of their own birth experiences and a sympathetic understanding of labour.

As time went on, women from outside the family were brought in. These were the early lay midwives, rewarded first with gifts, later by payment. They were the first professional birth attendants. Most of them were likely to have children of their own and they inevitably gained further knowledge of the process through constant observation and participation. They passed this knowledge on to each other from generation to generation in a tradition that has no parallel now.

So women in labour were surrounded by the familiar and the female. Men other than the father of the child were called in only if there was a dire emergency, an abnormal birth in which every conceivable effort on the part of mother and midwife to push and pull out the baby had failed. Then a man would be asked to use his strength and experience of foaling horses and lambing to help deliver a damaged child.

Even the advanced culture of ancient Greece and the development of medicine by men like Hippocrates revered the knowledge and status of women in childbirth, and stood by the order of women delivering babies in normal labours and men being called in to deal with abnormalities.

The first male physicians were priests. Midwives would ask for their assistance in difficult births. By the fourth century A.D., these doctor-priests were consulted for most abnormal births, and it became established that men would be present in cases where there were complications to delivery. This did not change until well into the sixteenth century.

It was the French surgeon Ambroise Paré who first described the introduction of foreign material into the delivery of children, when he recorded that by bringing out the legs of a child first, tying them with braid, and pulling hard, it was possible to deliver a child that could not be delivered head first. This was in 1551. Not long after, came the invention of obstetrical forceps. A step further than braid, forceps were used to clamp the baby's head while still in the birth canal, so the male physician, still the administrator in abnormal births, could then pull out the child by the head.

Forceps were invented in England by the Chamberlen family, accoucheurs and barber-surgeons. The first Chamberlen, William, came to England as a Huguenot refugee in 1569. His sons, Peter the elder and Peter the younger, attended the English court, and the queens of James I and Charles I as barber-surgeons and obstetricians, yet they were constantly in conflict with the College of Physicians because of alleged 'irregular practice', in other words using their primitive version of the modern forceps. Peter Chamberlen the younger lived from 1572 until 1626, practising as a surgeon and obstetrician, but it is thought that it was Peter the elder, who died in 1631, who first invented and used forceps.

By the late 1770s men and women birth attendants were quarrelling. Who was to conduct labour and delivery? The battle for status was on. Ancient tradition had always held that woman, with her superior knowledge and experience, was most qualified to attend normal deliveries. The man took his place in the event only when there was some obstacle to normal birth. But now that man was establishing his medical expertise, in an age when there were no female rights, he won the race for obstetrical superiority with his instruments, his booklearning and his dominant position in the social hierarchy. The battle became political.

Economic monopolization of medicine meant control over its institutional organizations, its theory, its practice, its profit and prestige. It still does. In fact even more so now that production of intricate, expensive scientific machinery has made obstetrical medicine a big-money industry in itself. The rise of male power in medicine began when the male physician started to serve the ruling classes.

It was the female healers who were of the people for the people. Their suppression began in medieval Europe. By the end of the fifteenth century midwives were often accused of being witches, and were hounded as such. Witches were hunted and burned from Germany, through Europe, to England. The so-called witches, for the most part, were lay healers, especially midwives. But they represented a political, religious and sexual threat to the Protestant and Catholic churches alike, as well as to the State which was, at that time, strongly aligned to organized religion. So midwives and women healers had little chance against the condemnation of the all-powerful male rulers of society. In the late fifteenth and early sixteenth centuries there were thousands and thousands of executions of these women in Europe, usually live burnings at the stake. For example, in the Bishopric of Trier, France, in 1585, two villages were left with only one female inhabitant each.

Male physicians supported this travesty of justice; '. . . Because the Medieval Church, with the support of kings, princes and secular authorities, controlled medical education and practice, the Inquisition from which [witch-hunts] developed constituted, among other things, an early instance of the "professional" repudiating the skills and interfering with the rights of the "non-professional" to minister to the poor'.[1]

It was, contrary to some beliefs, a well-organized, legal procedure. Witch-hunts were campaigns initiated, financed and executed by Church and State. There was a specific edict on the conduct of the witch-hunt, the *Malleus Maleficarum*,[2] or 'Hammer of Witches', written in 1484 by the Reverends Kramèr and Sprenger, priests of Pope Innocent VIII. The witch trials had to be initiated by either the Vicar (priest) or Judge of the County. Anyone suspected of being a witch or 'heretic' was to be reported immediately. Anyone failing to report a so-called witch faced excommunication from the Church and a long list of temporal punishments.

'Witchcraft' was never clearly defined, but it was a useful word to cover political subversion and any stand that a woman might make for her right to do as she wished and heal other women. Female healing was labelled heresy, lewdness and blasphemy. Midwives were accused of gross female sexuality, because they dealt in the care of female reproductive organs; they were accused of having 'magical' powers in the most demeaning, inaccurate and superstitious sense, simply because they were well versed in the healing properties of herbs, and used them medicinally.

The Church associated women with sex, and all pleasure in sex was condemned because it could only come from the Devil. Women as individuals were condemned out of hand in the *Hammer of Witches*, which says: 'When a woman thinks alone, she thinks evil.'

Yet 'witch-healers' were often the only general medical practitioners for working people who were bitterly afflicted with poverty and disease. The association of witch and midwife was inevitable. Kramer and Sprenger wrote: 'No one does more harm to the

1. Thomas Szasz, *The Manufacture of Madness*, London, 1973.
2. *Malleus Maleficarum* by Heinrich Kramer and James Sprenger, translated by Rev. Montague Summers, London, 1970.

Catholic Church than the midwife.' As we have seen from the history of the Chamberlen family, there was nothing in the Church's dogma which condemned medical care for the kings and nobles of the time. Male healing under the auspices of the monarchy was acceptable, female healing as part of the peasant culture was not.

There was total confusion between black magic, an illusory product of hysterical minds, and medicine. But many of the herbal remedies used then, are used now. Healers had pain-killers, digestive aids and anti-inflammatory agents. They used ergot for pain in labour, derivatives of which are used today, but this again was condemned by the Church because it was woman's duty to bring forth children in sorrow, religious punishment for Eve's original sin.

The midwife's work was based on belief in the evidence of the senses. She trusted, and the pregnant woman trusted, in her ability to find ways to deal with the hazards of pregnancy and childbirth. It was empirical medicine. The Church profoundly mistrusted the senses, and taught its followers to believe only in the non-material after-life. Hence, the midwife became the heretic. Paracelsus, now considered the father of pharmacology, burned his text on pharmaceuticals in 1527, confessing that he 'had learned from the Sorceress all he knew'.[1]

It was drugs that finally confirmed man's ringmaster role in obstetrics. The development of anaesthetics for relieving pain and man's exclusive legal right to dispense them made him the ruler of the childbed. Laughing gas, which we call nitrous oxide and is still used in delivery, was discovered in 1772 by Joseph Priestley and used for toothache. Seventy-five years later, American doctors found that ether had much the same effect as laughing gas, and by the middle of the nineteenth century it was being used as a labour anaesthetic both in England and America. Then a Scottish obstetrician, James Young Simpson, found chloroform knocked out his patients more efficiently and caused fewer nauseous side effects. Queen Victoria clinched the fashion for chloroform babies in 1853 by allowing herself to be anaesthetized by her physicians during the birth of Prince Leopold.

1. Barbara Ehrenreich and Deirdre English, *Witches, Midwives and Nurses*, London, 1974.

Seduced into oblivion, women quickly rejected the ministrations of familiar midwives in favour of doctors and drugs. Men were content. They made money from it, and the sense of power, too, is addictive. Midwives were ousted from their position because they could not legally use anaesthetizing agents. Their experience and training was only in childbirth, not in drugs, only of women and their bodies and their babies. Instruments, interference, medication had always been the province of men. Medicine was established as a profession, requiring university training. It was easy to bar women from practice. Women were precluded from Universities and the Royal College of Physicians. They could not qualify as doctors, and had been unable to since as far back as 1322, when the Faculty of Medicine at the University of Paris brought a woman doctor, Jacoba Felicie, to trial on charges of illegal practice, although, unlike most women healers then, she was literate and had received some formal training in medicine. Despite the fact that six witnesses claimed she had cured them, that testimony was used against her. The charge was that she, a woman, had dared to cure at all. It was a man's world. Then later, at the beginning of the twentieth century, as anaesthetics for delivery became fashionable, so doctors at delivery became fashionable too. Pregnant women, knowing very little about themselves and the nature of birth, seeking only relief from an experience they had been led to believe was fearful and uncontrollably painful, turned from nature to man.

As woman lost faith in herself, inevitably she lost faith in other women. The true value of the midwife was denigrated. Technology did nothing to help. Rather, it turned its own inventions into new myths. The myth of the infallible machine managed by the infallible man. Women's confidence has been undermined for so long, they have little experience of trusting themselves or each other. Men encouraged women to hand the responsibilities for safe birth to them. Men could manage the whole thing. They couldn't bring forth life, but they could direct it. They could control the event.

They moved on quickly from the discovery of chloroform. 1902: twilight sleep: morphine and scopolamine. A combination of heavy sedatives that induced a dreamy half-sleep somewhere between waking and unconsciousness. It obliterated the memory of sensation. You could have a baby without knowing anything about it, and women conditioned by ignorance could only welcome this as release from fear and pain.

In no time the difference between methods for normal and abnormal births, healthy and unhealthy pregnancies, smudged together. The physician was trained to deal with birth as an illness, to cope particularly with abnormalities. He preferred to operate from hospital rather than go to the woman in her home. Hospital delivery became the norm. The family bond of birth ritual has subsided with the advent of technology. As it is now, midwives in so-called developed countries all over the world are relegated to inferior positions in the medical hierarchy. They defer to the male physician, whether they are lay midwives or, as is normal in England, nurse-midwives, who do have the benefit of a medical training but are still only allowed to dispense a limited amount of drugs and are unable to perform any kind of surgery except for an occasional episiotomy (cutting the skin of the vaginal area before delivery) under the supervision of a doctor. The medical establishment is still structured around the supremacy of the male, even in the delicate area of childbirth.

I mistrust men as *sole* deliverers of my children. There are whole areas of female feeling that I doubt they understand. I see that a woman is more easily controlled and regimented in a sedated state, or unnaturally subdued by institutionalization. I do not see why it is so often considered essential to subdue a woman in labour. Deadening pain by artificial means is a modern obsession and through it we may lose the power of feeling. Are men so threatened by women's ability to bring life to fruition that they feel impelled to persuade her to dull her awareness of giving birth? It is extraordinary to realize how women have relinquished responsibility in birth, and how men have seized it. Authoritarianism often arises from fear that a greater authority will rise and strike. The chain of reaction is endless, unless we see what is happening and call a halt. Power need not be aggressive and I believe that human evolution can only come about through men and women understanding one another and working together, instead of each fighting for supremacy.

As it is, men have effectively shut women out from their own ritual and tried to obscure instinct with scientific expertise and machines. If you don't like the idea, you can be the one to change it, by the way you prepare for and go through your own Naturebirth.

Are Hospitals the Best Birthplaces?

Both sides of the Atlantic a woman is now expected to go to hospital to produce a baby. Very soon the National Health Service aims to see that every birth in the United Kingdom takes place in hospital. In America, in virtually all of the states, it is considered peculiar for a woman to reject the idea of hospital delivery, and although there are women gathering together to fight for their right to have a home delivery, minority groups are usually dismissed as eccentric.

In Britain the National Health Service offers free medical attention and dental service to pregnant women. In most countries a woman is expected to attend her local hospital or ante-natal clinic once a month during the third, fourth, fifth and sixth month. During the last three she may be asked to attend more often depending on results of blood-pressure checks, urine tests, weight gain and physical examination. During the ninth month it is expected that she attend at least once every two weeks.

If she is a private 'patient', her gynaecologist will tell her when to visit his office, or hospital. Welfare and National Health patients can expect a less personal contact. Over the course of a pregnancy they are likely to see many different doctors, sometimes students will attend for their lessons in obstetrics. It is virtually impossible to strike up a secure relationship with a member of the medical staff because the woman does not know who will deliver the baby, and seldom looks at the room where she will give birth. In most cases women don't see the midwife or the maternity ward unless permission is specifically requested. The father of the child is not often enough encouraged to be present at delivery, and if the woman is unmarried she may find her lover forcibly turned away, unless she has reached agreement with the hospital authorities beforehand.

Clinics usually mean waiting in line for between three and four hours. There is no provision made for domestic crisis, so if you miss one appointment you cannot make it for the next day. You have a file and a number and that is who you are.

Some hospitals run classes for relaxation. They usually suggest that a woman starts in the seventh month of pregnancy so that she attends at least eight sessions before the baby is born. In England, classes given for National Health patients are free, last for an hour and take place once a week. In effect, cost, location and technique vary from hospital to hospital. The times are awkward for most men to attend and very often there is no encouragement for men to participate. To tell the truth, I think I would find it hard to explore my sexual and spiritual experiences in a clinic. Remember birth is the only miracle which men and women are likely to experience directly. Since their sexuality initiated the miracle, why should so many hospitals effectively separate men and women at this time? Why should one of the most glorious things that ever happens to us be either dreadful or blank? Life stone cold dead. No feeling.

Twentieth-century woman is bred to have assembly-line babies. There are few exceptions that I know of. One of the few is London's Charing Cross Hospital, which goes further than most to encourage natural birth and the presence of fathers. England veers towards complete hospitalization of birth, and hospitals all over the world daily become more mechanized. In a handful of places in England there is a faint stirring of innovation, a recognition that there might be needs during birth which are not being met by hospitals. So the General Practitioners Units are appearing, to try to bridge the gap between mothers and professional obstetricians. These are flexible arrangements made by groups of G.P.s and hospitals, to enable a midwife to attend a woman, along with her own doctor, during her pregnancy, and then accompany her to hospital. This way the mother has familiar figures with her, has access to emergency facilities, and her own doctor retains care and responsibility during delivery, without hospital interference. Personal contact, established between the family, the doctor and the midwife in pregnancy, can then be maintained until after the birth. Not so in most cases. Sadly. Such facilities are still desperately inaccessible to most mothers.

Our hospitals are like factories, inhospitable, cold, but most of all quick. Quick efficient assembly-line babies born into sterility. Needles and blades and masks; pills, uniforms, no smell. 'Everything is done for you.' 'Here are your pills and here is your baby.' Scars on the bed in the head in the heart on the womb in the mind. 'Let me hold my baby.' 'Maybe maybe.'

Mothers do not behave in hospital as they do at home. A woman who is flat on her back and filled with drugs is much easier to handle than one who is up and doing. If you are not careful, once you are in hospital, you are down and out. Routine and hierarchy smother communication. The pharmacological management of labour is presumably easier for the medical profession because it does not have to take into account human emotions. Sedation is offered liberally, and eagerly accepted, to suppress the outward show of birth feelings. It is not socially acceptable to 'freak out', to display emotion. Mechanical routine cannot accept ecstasy. But every woman has a right to say 'no' to medication and 'no' to machines. Not every woman realizes she has this right, because she becomes intimidated by the institution.

Primitive women have various different ways of coping with the outrush of life. Historical evidence shows that since the beginning of recorded time, the natural position for women during birth for the expedient expulsion of the child, is upright—either standing, sitting, or crouching. Some, like the Hopje Indians, take to the mountains even now, others squat in the fields. My own instinct is to squat or crouch, at any rate for my head to be held higher than my abdominal area, so that I can see what's going on, stay in touch with the progress of my baby, and really help to push him out.

There is now evidence that what is called the 'lithotomy' position —back flat, legs in stirrups—which most hospitals and doctors prefer for delivery, does alter the normal fetal environment and obstruct the natural process of childbearing, making spontaneous birth more difficult or even impossible.

Although, having had babies, it seems again like the simplest common sense to me to be sitting up for labour and delivery, just because it's more comfortable and feels more natural—the word of a woman is hardly ever enough to get doctors to listen. They say they need facts not feelings. Well here are the facts, according to one report by the International Childbirth Education Association.[1]

It has been found that the lithotomy and dorsal (lying flat on your back) positions tend to:

1. affect adversely the mother's blood pressure, cardiac return and pulmonary ventilation;

1. Special Report, *The Cultural Warping of Childbirth, 1972*, by the International Childbirth Education Association, U.S.A., Vol. 11, Number 1, p. 21.
Flowers, C.: *Obstetric Analgesia and Anesthesia*, Hoeber, New York, 1967.
James, L. S.: 'The Effects of Pain Relief for Labor and Delivery on the Fetus and the Newborn', *Anesthesiology*, 21: 405, 1960.

2. decrease the normal intensity and efficiency of the contractions;
3. inhibit the mother's voluntary efforts to push her baby out spontaneously;
4. increase the need for forceps and increase the tractions necessary for a forceps extraction;
5. inhibit the spontaneous expulsion of the placenta which in turn increases the need for cord traction, forced expression or manual removal of the placenta—procedures which significantly increase the incidence of fetomaternal hemorrhage;
6. increase the need for episiotomy because of the increased tension on the pelvic floor and the stretching of the perineal tissue.

The sitting position is used as a general practice in the Netherlands, which has one of the lowest infant mortality rates in the world. The fact that combined use of both vacuum extractor and forceps in a delivery rarely exceeds 4 per cent of *all* births in that country, points to its advantages. In many American hospitals the incidence of forceps deliveries can be as high as 65 per cent.[1]

One of the more unpleasant 'accepted' practices in a normal hospital labour is for a woman to be subjected to rubber-fingered probing while she is trying to deal with contractions. Yet midwives are almost always able to judge the strength of uterine contractions and therefore the progress of the birth by putting a hand on the abdomen. Somehow institutionalization robs women of the courage to stop a man from sticking his finger up her vagina or her anus. If it were done in any other place by any other person it would be called indecent assault. To a labouring woman who does not want this intrusion, it may be the same invasion of privacy.

Shaving the pubic hair is an almost sadistic act which takes place in most hospitals. It is supposed to be for sanitary protection, because

1. International Childbirth Education Association Special Report, p. 22, Volume II, No. I, 1972.

Blankfield, A.: 'The Optimum Position for Childbirth', *Medical Journal*, Australia, 2: 666, 1965.

Howard, F. H.: 'Delivery in the Physiologic Position', *Obstetrics and Gynecology*, 11: 318, 1958.

Gritsiuk, I.: 'Position in Labor', *Obstetrics-Gynecology Observer*, September, 1968.

Newton, N. and Newton, M.: 'The Propped Position in Labor', *Obstetrics and Gynecology*, 15: 28, 1960.

hairs attract germs. But hair can be washed. And research involving 7,600 mothers[1] showed that there was slightly less infection among the women who were not shaved. Yet, often without the soothing froth of shaving cream, sometimes without even warm water, with only a scrub of soap and no lather, the hairs are torn from the most sensitive erogenous part of us. Even the upper part of the pubic hairline disappears, although there no one need look, nothing is hidden or about to emerge. But it will take weeks of scratchy ugliness to transform the stubble to softness again.

Another routine practice in most European hospitals, certainly English ones, is the administering of an enema during the early part of labour. An enema is given by a peculiarly uncomfortable instrument for the injection of liquid into the rectum. In other words, in the middle of a contraction, through which you are trying to breathe to the correct level and relax as comfortably as you can, someone comes along with a little device to stick up your anus and squirt soapy water into your back passage. It is unpleasant at the calmest of times, because you have to hold in the liquid until you can bear it no longer, usually timed by a nurse who will not let you run for the lavatory sooner than she says, then all hell breaks loose as your bowels erupt in protest.

The idea is to flush out anything which may be ejected involuntarily during the last stages of labour and when the pressure of delivery causes you to push. It is true that defecation during delivery may offend the sensibilities of the medical staff or indeed of the unprepared mother. Doctors also argue that there is a chance that your waste products loosened during delivery could be a source of infection.

Yet I found that at the beginning of labour for all three children I naturally emptied my bowels. One of the signs that I was really going into labour was a mild attack of diarrhea, which does everything the enema does, without the appalling discomfort. I understand from other women that this is quite usual in normal labour. I feel therefore that an enema is only warranted in cases of extreme impaction or constipation, and should not be given as a matter of routine.

Episiotomy, or 'surgical incision to enlarge the vaginal orifice' is

1. Burchell, R.: 'Predelivery Removal of Pubic Hair', *Obstetrics and Gynecology*, 24: 272, 1964.

now standard procedure in almost all hospital deliveries. One reason for doctors to perform an episiotomy is to avoid the danger of a jagged tear appearing between the vagina and the rectum. It may be quicker and easier to cut the skin of the perineum, but risks could be avoided by allowing the woman to sit up, so relieving the tension on her perineum and helping her to push the baby out herself. It is sometimes claimed that episiotomy reduces the chance of damage to a woman's pelvic floor, or neurological damage to the baby.[1] But in a normal labour, when the baby is full term and there is no sign of fetal distress, I could find no evidence to support this. If it is done to avoid a forceps delivery, so much the better. I'd certainly say cut my vagina before you put forceps to my baby's head. But again, it seems to be one of those things that doctors and midwives have become used to doing without enough thought as to whether the particular mother needs it, because it is a part of the routine.

It is the practice of many hospitals to take babies from their mothers immediately after birth. In America this is often to put them into artificial warming devices, which always carry a risk of breaking down. Yet the temperature of a healthy baby born to a relatively unmedicated mother should not drop if he is held in his mother's arms immediately.[2] Even clinical research demonstrates that hospital routine after birth seems to inhibit rather than encourage maternal response and nurturing. A 'controlled study' in America[3] suggests that 'the mother's increased sensitivity to her newborn infant during the first twenty-four hours following birth may be a biochemical mechanism which is not yet understood.' Not yet understood by whom? Hospitals perhaps. But certainly an aware woman who has borne a child knows that.

I was lucky enough to understand before going into labour with my second child that if you feel deeply enough, you can bend the rules and transform the environment. Going through the preparation detail by detail will show you how this can be managed, if you are unable to have your baby at home.

1. Butler, N.: 'A National Long Term Study of Perinatal Hazards', 6th World Congress, Federation of International Obstetricians and Gynecologists, 1970.

2. Dahm, L. and James, L.: 'Newborn Temperature: Heat Loss in the Delivery Room', *Pediatrics*, 49: 504, 1972.

3. Preface to the 4th edition of *Childbirth without Fear* by Dr Grantly Dick-Read, 1959.

Are Home Deliveries, Attended by Midwives, a Viable Alternative?

'*I am persuaded from long years of experience amongst women of many nationalities that good midwifery is essential for the true happiness of motherhood—that good midwifery is the birth of a baby in a manner nearest to the natural law and design.*'[1]

Having your baby at home has become something extraordinary, an idea viewed with suspicion. It is a mark of the speed at which our lives and styles have changed. Twenty years ago the normal thing to do was to have your baby at home. My mother had both her children at home. Most women did. Even in the late fifties more than half the children in England were born at home. Now we have a six per cent rate of home deliveries because hospital has become *the* place to bear a child.

Part of the reason for this is the attitude which has taken hold, that giving birth is automatically treated as a sickness, that we need the 'safety' of medicines and mechanization in order to deliver our children. Our own bodies have ceased to provide a sense of security to most of the people of the second half of the twentieth century. When childbirth is presented as an abnormal condition, those who are not in the habit of questioning assumptions will simply accept them. Part of the confusion that arises in peoples' minds about childbirth and its difficulties lies in the fact that so little distinction is made between 'normal' and 'abnormal' birth. This means that most of us are unaware of the differences when we should be acutely aware of them.

When trying to make a decision as to whether you have your baby at home or in hospital, you have to know whether you or the baby are at risk, both during pregnancy and delivery. A pregnancy with known abnormalities, obstetrical complications, or even a hint of possible difficulty needs quite different attention to that given a woman in a completely normal healthy pregnancy. Complications should undoubtedly be watched over by those trained to deal with complications, and such a pregnancy will probably require specialized care at birth. The woman is as much a patient then as she is *not* in the circumstances of normal pregnancy and birth.

1. *Childbirth without Fear* by Grantly Dick-Read, London, 1942.

An abnormal pregnancy leading to an abnormal delivery can be caused by physiological or anatomical abnormality within the mother, or the possibility of the fetus itself being unhealthy. Chronic forms of maternal diseases, such as diabetes, abnormalities of the thyroid or kidneys or raised blood pressure would all need careful management. So also would a pregnancy during which a woman has vaginal bleeding, when twins or a multiple birth is expected, when a woman is found to belong to the Rhesus negative blood group, when she is a junkie, or if she has an extremely small pelvis in relation to the size of the baby, or if she has had a previous Caesarean section.

Such abnormalities occur only during about 30 per cent of births. A pregnancy without signs of complication has every chance of continuing that way, so that a healthy woman should bear a healthy child after a normal labour, and in more than 70 per cent of pregnancies the antenatal period and confinement *are* completely normal.[1]

The problem is that there is always an element of surprise to be taken into consideration. There is a small percentage of deliveries, one that doctors suggest cannot be definitively estimated, in which unforeseen complications could arise. Doctors, obstetricians, take care of the woman in labour. They are there to see that nothing goes wrong, and approach birth from that point, so that for most doctors the risks to home delivery are that there will not be adequate means with which to treat a woman.

Yet according to Professor G. J. Kloosterman, head of obstetrics and gynaecology at one of Amsterdam's leading hospitals, it is his experience that two thirds of all pregnant women, having been checked first for risk of any kind, would deliver naturally and need only be attended by midwives, and that during delivery only between 3 per cent and 5 per cent of healthy women would ever require consultation with a doctor.[2] Holland has a consistently low infant mortality rate, 11·1 per cent in 1971, compared to 18·5 per cent in the States during the same year, and a consistently high rate of successful home deliveries. Kloosterman points out that in a group of 20,000 deliveries by midwives there was not one case in which an obstetrician rather than a midwife was needed.

1. *Gynaecology* by Derek Llewellyn Jones, M.D., London, 1971.
2. Speech at the 50th anniversary of the International Confederation of Midwives, U.S.A., 1972.

I can see why the medical establishment has become so entrenched in its dismissive attitude to home delivery, and the safety of the woman giving birth is an honourable motive. The mistake seems to me to be in assuming that a *healthy* woman is any safer in hospital than out of it. Woman should be given more credit for being able to handle the experience herself, and giving birth in her own home might make it more familiar, more harmonious, relaxing, and therefore, in a normal delivery, probably much easier. In being offered the opportunity of honouring her own birthright, perhaps a woman who has never considered the subject before, might shake herself free of conditioning and rise to the challenge. Dutch obstetricians underline the fact that when a labour is normal and allowed to proceed in an unhurried way, the unexpected emergencies rarely occur.[1] Professor Kloosterman goes so far as to say that a very healthy woman *is* sometimes better off at home.

Holland's maternal mortality rate is, like the infant mortality rate, very low in comparison to most Western countries. In 1974 it was 0·4 per 10,000 births, whereas in Britain in 1970, about one woman in every 6,600 died in childbirth. So there you have a country in which more than half the babies are born at home, with midwives to assist, and a lower rate of mother and child mortality than either the United Kingdom or the United States, both of which have almost 100 per cent institutionalization of births. So who is to say with absolute authority that a hospital delivery is necessarily 'safer' than a home delivery for a healthy woman?

Home deliveries could and should be a realistic choice for the majority of healthy women who bear healthy children. It is only just beginning to be so again in my country, England, and in America. What we really need is a properly developed service for home deliveries. England's answer to sudden emergencies during home births was the Flying Squad. I say was, because these specially equipped, obstetrician-accompanied ambulances used to be on call for all domiciliary midwives, but now, with the decline of domiciliary midwifery, they scarcely exist. If they were revived in Britain and innovated in America, it would eliminate virtually all the element of risk taken on when you choose a home delivery. Encouraging women to believe in and to become midwives would help develop everybody's trust in the

1. I.C.E.A. News, p. 15, *The Cultural Warping of Childbirth*, U.S.A., 1972.

midwife's ability to fulfil her role with responsibility, in keeping with her ancient tradition. More training and more opportunities could be made available and easily accessible for women interested in continuing that tradition, or reviving it to fit our times.

But the facts of the matter are that most midwives in England who receive the required two to three years medical training, either solely in midwifery, or as nurses first, work in hospitals. Only about six thousand out of the seventy thousand midwives in the United Kingdom work 'on the district'. In other words they are assigned a particular area by local health authorities, who pay them, and only then can they attend home births in that district. Very few doctors want to attend home births because they have so little time. Home deliveries, city or country, are discouraged by most of the medical profession, for whom they constitute extra work in an already over-burdened schedule. In America you can pay a great deal of money for an obstetrician to attend your delivery, but he will do so in his hospital, where he has all his props. In England you can also pay a private doctor or consultant to attend you but the laws are different, and if he accepts payment from you on the understanding that you want a home delivery, then he attends you at the place of your choosing. If you are a National Health patient, in which case the Government is paying the doctor to provide a service, you are not employing him, then he can and will refuse to attend you if it is inconvenient. Therefore you usually have to pay for a home delivery, although it is probably less than half the sum you would have to pay to see a specialist throughout pregnancy, and be delivered at his hospital.

Until about ten years ago it was more or less assumed in the United Kingdom that a woman would have her first baby in hospital and her second or third at home. Now the large, modern hospitals full of equipment are drawing mothers towards institutionalized deliveries, even if the woman only stays the minimum forty-eight hours, instead of the advised six to ten days after a first baby, or two days after subsequent children. In the United States the usual period of confinement is about five days. Another of the weird things that happens to women in hospital is that they tend to believe they *have* to stay in hospital for the advised ten days, when in actual fact you can dismiss yourself from a hospital at any time and are not bound to accept the suggestions of the staff. This could be because such suggestions usually sound more like orders than advice.

Second, third, fourth and fifth babies as a general rule are far less susceptible to risk in terms of obstetric complications than the first and the sixth. For the first, sixth and later babies doctors invariably try to hospitalize a woman if there is any reasonable medical doubt that labour will not follow a normal course. They also seem to consider a woman suspiciously if she is over thirty-three, after which ancient age she may be viewed as beyond the pale as far as having babies is concerned. Clearly if you haven't had a baby until then, your bones may have begun to set too much, limbs could have become too creaky, or skin too taut to encompass easily the growth of a child within. But I seriously doubt that a healthy, relaxed woman whose body is in good physical shape, should have any more difficulty having her baby at home if she is over thirty-three; especially if she has already borne children.

Remember that for a home birth you must have a midwife, and the problem is that in most places domiciliary midwifery is a dying profession. Great Britain and the European countries have their ancient and respected tradition of lay midwifery. But it has taken a disastrous tumble in the last few years. Now a midwife must have a formal medical training, and usually works in a hospital. America has practically no tradition of female lay healing because it was uprooted so early in the nation's history. When the first settlers arrived in the States, the women brought their healing secrets too, among them the timeless rites of birthing. By the beginning of the twentieth century those rites and the women who performed them had been completely discredited, and the role of lay midwife evaporated in the harsh glare of approaching technology.

As the United States emerged as the industrial leader of the world, money poured into the coffers of an elite group of male medical practitioners, known then as 'the regulars', to differentiate them from the women healers, banned from medical faculties, who were called the 'irregulars'. By 1830, thirteen States had passed medical licensing laws outlawing 'irregular' practices, one of which was midwifery, and establishing 'regulars', men, as the only legal healers. By 1848 male doctors had their first national organization, called the American Medical Association. By 1903, millions of dollars were flowing into the medical schools. The regular doctor was a professional. He was paid, and he had access to the mystique of science. In state after state tough new licensing laws were passed to seal the doctors' monopoly on medical practice, yet in 1910 about 50 per cent of babies were still being delivered by midwives. This was intolerable to male obstetricians. They attacked. Midwives were proclaimed hopelessly dirty, ignorant and incompetent. They were specifically blamed for uterine infections and neonatal ophthalmia, which is the blindness in babies caused by parental infection with gonorrhea. Despite the fact that Professor John Hopkins' survey in 1912 indicated that doctors were in fact *less* efficient than midwives because they were not only unreliable in preventing disease but also too ready to use surgical techniques which endangered mother and child, it was the doctors who had the *power*. Under pressure from this powerful rather than competent group, the male medical profession, even more states passed laws making midwifery illegal and restricting the practice of obstetrics to doctors.

The role of women in healing has been dramatically and tragically quashed, and the last few years of woman's liberation has done little to even the odds in the medical profession. Ninety-three per cent of doctors in the United States are men. In England the figure stands at 76 per cent. Lower, but hardly fifty-fifty. Almost all the top directors and administrators of health institutions in Britain and America are men. Very few women are gynaecologists or obstetricians, despite the fact that these two professions deal solely with childbirth and diseases related to the female reproductive function. Seventy per cent of health workers in the States are women, but they are *workers* not specialists.[1] Even nurses, who form the backbone of the medical profession, are ancillary workers in relation to doctors. (Ancillary is taken from the Latin word 'ancilla' which means maidservant.) Just as women in labour and delivery are taught that 'doctor knows best', so too are nurses still the lower echelon of the medical hierarchy. In America neither nurses nor nurse-midwives are able to administer medication without being under orders from a doctor. So man has science with which to work and mystify. Woman is almost always subservient to the myth of man and science.

The midwife in America still has no recognized status unless she is a nurse-midwife and works within the hospital regime. A midwife

1. *A History of Women Healers* by Barbara Ehrenreich and Deirdre English, p. 1, 1974, Compendium Press, England; Feminist Press, U.S.A.

wanting to attend a home birth has no legal right to even carry the things she may need for delivery, no right to ask for payment or be paid for her services, no obstetrical back-up should there be an emergency. A woman who wants to be a midwife is only considered 'qualified' if she has been certified by the state as having attended a training college. Even then nurse-midwives cannot act without the supervision of a doctor, cannot prescribe or give drugs, cannot use forceps or perform surgery. In England the situation is a little better in that midwives do administer drugs in limited doses and do perform episiotomies, but if it is a home delivery, the doctor must be on call at all times, even if he is not present.

There are no longer any lay midwives in England as there were at the beginning of this century. The traditional midwife, handing down her knowledge by word of mouth, schooled in the lessons of childbirth through her own experience, no longer exists now that all midwives must first be nurses, or have fulfilled the statutory two years of formal medical training. However, it is at least still possible to find women who will attend to you at home in England. Although it is increasingly difficult to find midwives willing to go 'on the district' there is a new breed of young women, particularly in London, who cannot tolerate working within the regimented routine of hospital but sense the need to give women the opportunity of having their children at home.

In America there are a few small programmes, organized by nurse-midwives, which cater for women who want home deliveries in rural areas. The first of its kind began in Kentucky in 1929 as a privately funded, non-profit-making mobile unit, designed to meet the needs of mothers and babies in the Kentucky mountains and staffed by nurse-midwives who travelled by jeep within a five-mile radius. But now the service only covers pre-natal check-ups and all the babies are delivered in hospital. One of the reasons for this is that not even nurse-midwives can get any back-up service from doctors or hospitals for home deliveries. There is no available ambulance or medical equipment for the midwife even in emergency, and insurance companies will not cover home deliveries. You can only be insured for a hospital birth.

In New York, midwifery training was first introduced in 1931 by the Maternity Center Association, and is taught in various programmes around America, although there are still only about 1,500 practising midwives who are certified through this system. Most of them either get married and stop working, or go into teaching. Only a handful of them will dare to attend home deliveries since in almost all cases it puts them at personal risk. A 'qualified' nurse-midwife is first trained as a nurse and then acquires the further skills of being able to provide prenatal care, care during birth, and care of mother and child after birth. The catch is that this training and skill can only be put to use under the supervision of a physician and in the U.S.A. male obstetricians work from hospitals.

One Center in California, set up by women to give prenatal care to women wanting home deliveries, the Santa Cruz Birth Center, was raided by the police in March, 1974. Although they have been arraigned, the midwives have not yet been brought to trial. Midwifery was made non-legal in California as far back as 1949, when the provision for licensing midwives was revoked. Despite the State's rural communities' desire to find an alternative to hospitalization through home deliveries, it has been a desperate battle to change the law. California State Senator Anthony Beleinson introduced a bill in the State legislature to authorize the practice of nurse-midwifery in hospitals. The bill, put before the Assembly Health Committee, was opposed by the California Medical Association and the State Board of Medical Examiners, in spite of the fact that there are many obstetrician-gynaecologists who now advocate the training and licensing of nurse-midwives to supervise uncomplicated births. It was eventually passed in 1975.

The struggle to legalize domiciliary midwifery is obviously crucial to the whole question of home delivery, so also is the need to elevate the midwives' status from the level of inferior assistant and to encourage more women into domiciliary midwifery. Women should at least be allowed a choice in whether they have their children at home or in hospital, but lack of available home care makes the balance of alternatives unequal.

3

The Mechanization of Birth

The Mechanics of Pregnancy

Technology's gallop into the machine age is transforming pregnancy and labour from processes directed by nature to exercises in mechanical research. It is a feat of modern medicine to be able to monitor the progress of a fetus inside a woman at virtually every stage of pregnancy, and so avoid perhaps some of the reasons for miscarriage, premature birth and damaged children. However, I do find it disturbing that women are now being encouraged to rely solely on hospitals and drugs to get them through labour, rather than learning to understand their own bodies; and those women who do discover some medical reason to have their baby's development monitored or induced are given little or no information about the machines to which their bodies are subjected.

A new science has grown up around the unborn child called 'fetal' medicine. But at the moment it is still a science for scientists and doctors, not for the women without whom it would not exist. Most doctors have forgotten how to communicate and few women want to become simply numbers in a statistic, or cases in a textbook of obstetrics, they want to be taken into account as human beings, they want to know why doctors are putting their bodies through the tests they do now, and for what reason their womb-life needs observing. It is not good enough to produce a machine without a reason. Mechanical devices have sprung up like mushrooms in the ante-natal clinics and the delivery rooms. Technology has changed maternity so fast that the women going through it understand practically nothing of what is happening.

So if doctors are not going to make it their policy to tell us how and why they have mechanized birth, we are going to have to find out for ourselves. I tracked down as many methods and machines as I could, but came away from the research feeling that doctors themselves are so divided in their opinions and experience of these new techniques, that any woman seeking information from more than one doctor or hospital may come away with conflicting evidence. This is why searching out a sympathetic and understanding doctor to guide your pregnancy is so important. It is unfortunately true that many male gynaecologists and obstetricians have a tendency to think women know nothing about themselves, let alone about themselves pregnant. So while they're out there cracking the mysteries of our infants' hidden behaviour in the womb, forgetting that we might be feeling something they could learn from, they'd like us to be quiet, lie still, and not ask questions. Don't you remember that saying, 'Ask no questions, and you'll get no lies'? Well, I feel it's true of modern medicine, and most men of medicine have also lost sight of the fact that a woman might deeply resent the impersonal disinterested way in which she is so often treated when she wants information.

Machines have been introduced in pregnancy to try to pick up the baby's distress signals and help man figure out what is happening to the child in the woman. Yet I think only a small proportion of the medical profession is aware of how hopelessly intimidated some women are by machinery, especially during the illogical moodiness of pregnancy. To me at any rate, machines can represent authority and masculinity in its most threatening form, and if I have to be confronted with them, I want to know how they work, why they are being used on me and my baby, and what effect they may have on the metabolism of either one of us. If more doctors were ready to explain these things to mothers, there might not be such immediate suspicion, if not antipathy, between mother and machine as now certainly exists.

The moment of birth is supposedly the most dangerous of our lives and more babies die in the seven days after birth than in the seven following years, but it is also true that the womb is a risky place to be. The fetal environment has built-in hazards of its own. It is unfortunately true that in Britain alone one birth in every eighty is a stillbirth, and one baby out of every forty is likely to have a gross abnormality. There are about one million births a year but over twenty thousand stillbirths and neonatal deaths.[1]

A bad, or inefficiently functioning, uterine environment can cause a high percentage of the damage sustained by children before they are born. At least 80 per cent of the children born mentally handicapped each year have no hereditary reason for the defect,[2] which means a major proportion occur in the womb, and could possibly be prevented through efficient ante-natal care, not only careful checking by doctors, but personal care, preparation and protection by each woman for her unborn.

Machinery is now a part of pregnancy and its arrival has had some extraordinary advantages and some hair-raising disadvantages. Monitoring the early life and progress of the fetus in the womb and the state of the mother has given doctors a chance to detect the first signs of dangers like toxemia. It is also supposedly possible to determine the exact age of a fetus, and there is a technical method by which abnormalities in an embryo can sometimes be spotted very early in pregnancy, which may avoid unnecessary bearing of seriously handicapped children. However, the disadvantage to this is that intervention can, and occasionally does, cause miscarriage, and one gynaecologist has been quoted as saying that in one year of using this method, on the grounds of suspected mongolism, six of the test cases resulted in terminated pregnancies where the fetus was afterwards found to show no indication of mongolism.[3] So there are inherent dangers in the very sophistication of the tools now being used to detect danger. Since the for and against of the matter could be a question of life and death, let us at least make our decisions knowing the facts.

AMNIOCENTESIS

This is the process of taking a sample of the amniotic fluid surrounding the fetus. It is a particularly significant achievement in that it provides a means of ascertaining the possibility of mongolism, or what is called Down's Syndrome. In early pregnancy, between twelve and twenty weeks, the fetus begins shedding some of its cells

1. G. S. Dawes, 'Hazards of Birth', p. 133, *Human Reproduction: from the Science Journal*, London, 1971.
2. 'The Unborn Baby as Patient' by Ruth Inglis, *Nova*, p. 81, September, 1972.
3. *Ibid.*

into the amniotic fluid. A needle passing through the mother's abdominal wall can collect some of these cells, and in 80 per cent of all cases a culture can be grown from them in a laboratory. Then the chromosomes in a cell are counted. If there is one particular chromosome extra then there is a very real possibility of mongolism existing in the unborn child. Women over forty are those most likely to bear mongoloid children, but since the extra chromosome is not a definitive prediction of the degree of handicap, mothers of this age-group very often decide to keep their babies on the chance the child will be normal.

One of the setbacks of any medicine of interference is that it may spark off adverse reaction in the delicately balanced natural chemistry of the body. In this case it is important that women who want to take the test be aware that it might also cause miscarriage, which is why some doctors are reluctant to do it in the first three vulnerable months of pregnancy.

It seems to be much safer to perform tests on the amniotic fluid later in pregnancy and they are often used to assess Rhesus disease. Using amniocentesis, a doctor can judge whether the baby's condition is serious enough to warrant an intra-uterine blood transfusion, which is a complicated operation, not lightly undertaken.

One of the greatest fears doctors have about the unborn child is that its development may fall off rapidly in the last three months of pregnancy. When this does happen the babies are called 'small for dates', and one of the most common causes of this is that the blood from the placenta seems to be nourishing the baby inadequately. It can cause serious neurological damage to the unborn child, although in the less severe cases the baby may be born very underweight, but will respond to post-natal care.

Some of these babies do not grow normally, some thrive after birth. The dilemma lies in whether to induce early once you know the baby is small. The levels of certain substances in the blood serum of the mother (oestriol, placental lactogens) are also being tested in certain research centres as possible indicators of this trouble; and this method will probably spread.

If you are in any doubt about the health of your unborn baby, check with your doctor. The Royal College of Obstetricians and Gynaecologists in London issued a book called *Methods for Monitor-*

ing the Fetus in Pregnancy and Labour in October, 1971. On the subject of amniocentesis it cautiously warns:

'Amniocentesis is a safe procedure in skilled hands when the placenta is localized and aseptic techniques are used, but there is always a risk, and the value of the information that can be gained must be carefully balanced against the risk of this procedure in each individual patient.'

FETAL BLOOD SAMPLING

This is another way of checking the health of the unborn child. It is done by taking a small amount of blood from the scalp of the child during labour. This was first tested in 1962 by a German doctor and is now being used in Britain. King's College Hospital, London, a large teaching hospital equipped with all the latest machinery of birth, are now taking samplings of unborn babies regularly. The method is used particularly in the case of diabetic mothers to try and find out why the babies of diabetics have a tendency to die quickly in the last few weeks of pregnancy. So far this has been a mystery to doctors, and they are hoping blood sampling may help solve it, or at least give a clue as to what could be done to prevent the disease which obviously affects the child. If the fetus is in any trouble from oxygen starvation or other types of threatened last-minute asphyxiation, a blood sample will, according to Professor Beard, formerly an obstetrician of King's College Hospital, now at St Mary's Hospital Medical School, London, spell out the distress as clearly as any telegram.

ABDOMINAL FETAL ELECTROCARDIOGRAPH

This can be used from the twentieth week of pregnancy onwards to monitor the fetal heartbeat and study the progress and well-being of the fetus. Electrodes are attached to the mother's stomach near the baby's head and buttocks and the fetal heartbeats are amplified. The mother and supervising doctor are in a small sound-proof room, so that they can hear the exaggerated beat of the baby's heart as it comes through the machine and the rate of beat is then monitored by the electrocardiograph printing out a graph. This helps to assess maturity and position of fetus and placenta. It is used in labour as well as pregnancy. Normally a baby's heartbeat is twice as fast as its mother's, but this electrocardiograph shows that in labour his heart can beat wildly fast or quite slowly, according to how the extraordinary stress is put on him as labour takes its toll. Any deviation from the normal pattern either during pregnancy or labour would be picked up immediately and translated onto the graph.

In the United States the Fetal Heart Monitor is a similar device used in labour, a boxlike machine with long heavy straps that encircle the woman's abdomen and record internal vibrations. The strap around the upper abdomen has a pressure gauge which records uterine contractions; the lower strap holds an ultrasonic transducer which records the baby's heart rate. Both are connected to a machine that translates this information onto a long roll of paper like a chart of brainwave patterns.

The machine is so sensitive it may pick up irrelevant vibration, possibly from the mother's intestines and circulation, in which case doctors are not getting the information they need and would switch to internal monitoring by putting a plastic catheter up through the vagina and into the cervix, attaching it by a clip or screw to electrodes which are then fastened to the scalp of the baby trying to get through the birth canal. The fetal heartbeat is picked up best if the mother is flat on her back and immobile. She will probably also be hooked up to an intravenous drip of synthesized hormones to stimulate and control labour—and since it is vital to keep a check on blood pressure control under such conditions, there could also be a permanent blood-pressure monitor as well—either a technical device attached constantly, or an attendant to do it manually.

Note: A normal fetal heartbeat is between 120 and 160 beats per minute; above 160 indicates the child is in distress and possible danger and that something should be done about it; below 100 should be taken as a warning signal.

ABDOMINAL DECOMPRESSION MACHINE

This was invented in South Africa by Professor Ockert Heyns at Witwatersrand University, as a way of relieving some of the discomfort of pregnancy and labour for a woman and increasing the oxygen supply to the baby. It is a complex mechanical device into which a woman has to be strapped bodily. Made of PVC, the air-tight suit has a fibreglass dome which goes over the woman's belly. Complaints from women who have tried it are that it makes them feel dizzy and claustrophobic. Others say it relieves pressure aches and pains, particularly back-ache during pregnancy, and it is supposed to reduce the extreme pressure of contractions.

Once inside the PVC casing, which covers you from chest to thighs, pressure inside is reduced so that atmospheric pressure on the anterior abdominal wall is reduced, and this relieves pressure on the uterus. The release and return of pressure is designed to help the maternal flow of blood and improve circulation to the placenta and so to the baby.

Professor Heyns' claim was that research showed that babies born to women who had been using his machine were often brighter and more intelligent than others, because a better oxygen supply to the unborn baby helped in the development of the more sophisticated brain cells towards the end of pregnancy. Although there is great contention of this view, particularly by doctors from other countries, the Decompression machine has been used outside South Africa, and by 1968 it was being used in thirty-five different hospitals under Britain's National Health Service, especially for women with toxemia.

The impressive results recorded by Professor Heyns and J. A. Blecher, working on this in South Africa, do not seem to have been repeated in Britain.[1] But Heyns and Blecher maintain there was some improvement in 80 per cent of their toxemia cases, and a 12 per cent infant mortality rate against 28 per cent in patients treated with drugs.

ULTRASOUND MACHINE

This emits ultrasonic waves which are used to find out whether a baby is growing properly in the womb, by measuring the diameter of its head. Ultrasound means literally 'beyond the range of human ear'. Originally developed to track submarines during the Second World War, it is now used to track babies. The machine bombards the

1. *Pregnancy* by Gordon Bourne, F.R.C.S., F.R.C.O.G., p. 251, Cassells, London, 1972.

human body with sound pulses at frequencies pitched so high the human ear cannot hear them. There may be up to one thousand pulses a second, and their echoes from within the body are used by doctors to build up a picture on a screen similar to that of a television set. A graph of the baby's head size is drawn each week, and if the growth seems slow the obstetrician will be on the alert.

There are several types of this machine which measure various features of the unborn child as well as being able to give absolute confirmation of pregnancy in the early weeks. They measure the size of the baby's head, show the position of the placenta, record the fetal heartbeat and reveal one kind of tumour in the womb. It is now also being used during labour, if the baby seems to be small, your dates are in question, the baby's heartbeat faltering, or there is any reason to be on the lookout for distress signals.

You have to lie flat on your back, abdomen bared and well rubbed with oil. The 'eye' of the machine then goes backwards and forwards over your abdomen sending sound waves through its walls and through those of the uterus, which then relay their message onto the screen.

The most obvious procedure with which to compare it is X-ray, except that it does not use radiation as that is known to be harmful to the unborn baby. In fact ultrasound machines are really used instead of X-rays since they are supposedly safer, but fulfil approximately the same function. The machine is expensive. It costs £15,000 and was first used in pregnancy by Ian Donald in Glasgow in 1959. Now ultrasound is used routinely in normal as well as abnormal pregnancy and labour. A survey done by a market research company in Massachusetts shows, says the director, William Sullivan, that an estimated 75 to 80 per cent of women in America are tested by ultrasonic techniques. It was originally intended to help doctors detect the presence of diseases like tumours, not necessarily in pregnancy, much sooner than the conventional methods. The machine enables doctors to distinguish bone from soft tissues and organs.

When it was first brought into use it was discovered to be ideal for detecting the fetal heartbeat and monitoring the function of the heart during early pregnancy, but the medical press criticized its being used in attempts to scan the inside of an adult's head. Presumably doctors were in such cases looking for brain tumours. There is certainly some doubt in my mind as to why it should be considered irresponsible to scan the inside of an adult human head, but perfectly all right to expose the delicate, still-forming tissues of an unborn baby's brain to such high-frequency sounds.

There have been queries about possible damage to chromosomes, and although the general conclusion is that there is no chromosomal harm, certain doctors involved in the study of ultrasound admit there could be other factors which could cause damage in other ways. In a study of chick embryos subjected to ultrasound they found clumping of red blood cells, minute blood clots which slow down the flow of blood and could damage the rapidly developing tissues. The researchers say that there may be factors which set 'a safety limit to ultrasonic power level below that at which chromosomal damage occurs and that absence of such damage should not be relied on as a measure of safety'.[1]

Researchers in Japan are blaming the ultrasound machine—they use the Doppler, although the machines all have the same function— for tragically deformed babies. They believe it can cause birth defects—brain damage, deformity of limbs, jaws and genital organs, cleft palates.

Dr Tetsuya Shimizu, Professor of Gynaecology and Obstetrics at Hokkaido University, Sapporo, Japan, is head of the research team which first made public these findings in the spring of 1973. He says: 'Our research indicates that ultrasonic machines can cause thalidomide-like deformities in the fetus if done during the first three months of pregnancy. A warning from the Japan Association of Maternal Welfare in Tokyo has gone out to every doctor in Japan to stop using the machines during the first three months.'

Dr Shimizu, who studied in the States at Washington University, Seattle, on a Rockefeller Foundation scholarship, began his experiments in June 1972. He found that, using white mice for the tests, in those exposed to the Doppler (ultrasound) machines there was a dramatic increase in miscarriages and stillbirths. On the basis of this, the Japanese Ministry of Education co-sponsored an immediate second experiment, which confirmed the findings of the first. Shimizu

1. *British Medical Journal*, 30th September, 1972, p. 797. 'Effect of Ultrasound on Chromosomes of Lymphocyte Cultures' by U. Abdulla, D. Talbert, D. M. Lucas, M. Mullarkey.

claims that the machine has a disruptive effect on forming bone and tissue. His work is published in Japan and West Germany.

If studies are still being done on the validity and safety of ultrasonic machines during pregnancy, it indicates that doctors and scientists still don't know the exact effects of ultrasonic waves on the human embryo. Yet these machines have been in general use all over the world for more than ten years, scanning babies which may be developing quite normally without any need for this highly sophisticated form of diagnosis.

If there is any question of dangerous side-effects, testing with ultrasound or any other mechanical means in healthy pregnancies and normal labours definitely raises an issue of responsibility. If you encounter any one of these preceding techniques, find out exactly why it is being suggested you use it, what effect it is likely to have, and if there is any other means by which the same results might be achieved.

Note on X-rays

There's a certain amount of confusion about whether a woman is right to avoid being X-rayed while she is pregnant. Some hospitals scorn such fears and actually persuade people into the X-ray room in order to photograph the exact position of the baby, etc. You could also come in for an X-ray for possible broken bones. Make sure the doctors know you are pregnant and that you want to avoid excessive exposure to X-rays. Many doctors are now reluctant to X-ray even in second half of the period cycle, in case of pregnancy. Early in pregnancy they may kill the fetus; a little later they can deform it; and even later in pregnancy, when the child is formed, it may slightly increase his chance of developing leukemia or some other form of cancer in childhood.[1]

*   *   *

1. *Birth of a Baby*, The Marshall Cavendish Learning System: *Man and Medicine*, p. 39, London, 1969.

The Mechanics of Labour: Pain and Painkillers

It is important to remember that everyone has a different threshold of pain, and response to it. Some of us can tolerate more discomfort than others. Certain women seem to be better equipped to handle intense sensation, either by nature, environment or life-style. Others are conditioned to expect, if not to want, the edge taken off extreme feelings. Birth particularly, and its pangs, seems to assail women to various degrees and with broadly varying effects. There are vague guidelines as to who might feel more uncomfortable during labour than others. For instance, a woman with a very narrow pelvis is likely to have more difficulty producing a child than a wide-hipped woman. But it doesn't necessarily follow, and just as some large women have small babies after painful labours, so also some small women deliver large babies easily.

I think it was pain I felt in labour, anyway the first time. After the second, prepared, birth I felt that I could actually manage my response to the strangeness, the unaccustomed, unfamiliar wrench of contractions, and that in some way altered the concept of labour being 'painful'. But of course we all experience events differently. We use words to try to record and recall experiences, but are limited by language. Pain is experienced subjectively. We do not really know if our level of tolerance is dependent on state of mind, physiological make-up, or even just the time of day. Biologically it is a warning signal demanding a response from the organism experiencing it, to do something. Preparation gives you a choice. You can either freak out and wail. Or you can use your technique of breathing to help you relax and centre yourself. Psychologically, most people's responses to pain seem to be conditioned by lack of knowledge, which leads to fear which leads to tension which then aggravates pain. Particularly in labour, when the most important thing is that the only contracting part of you is the womb. It might sound complicated but it isn't really. The more you know, the less you fear and the less it hurts.

All sedating or painkilling drugs likely to be offered you in labour 'cross' the placenta and reach the baby with the same kind of depressant effect on his system that it has on yours. My feeling is that if you can do without any drugs, all the better for you and the baby. But I think it's important to reiterate the fact that the course of any labour is unpredictable. If you find you really want something to help you, beyond your breathing pattern and your own strength, then don't feel guilty about it afterwards. Don't feel inadequate. There is no blame. There is simply your labour and how you deal with it. The point to being prepared is that it is, if you want to try, much easier to deal with contractions without drugs. Understanding that pain is not unendurable, and can be dealt with, lessens its shock effect. When a woman is dozey from sedation, it is far harder for her to stay in touch with her labour. It is much more likely that she will willingly hand herself over to others. Succumbing to a drugged labour could make all the difference in the quality of your giving birth; could make the difference between it being a nightmarish haze and an exalting experience.

The medical view of childbirth seems to be that pain is inevitable. If you surrender yourself totally to the medical establishment to have your baby, then it is probable that you will be expected to want to dull your feelings. Apart from enlightened exceptions, the medical equation is: labour = pain = painkillers. Kill pain. What with? Drugs. What kind of drugs? Well, sorting that one out is like trying to walk through a maze blindfold. Drugs which relieve anxiety and tension, which numb pain, which kill pain, which make you sleepy, sick, oblivious, euphoric, stupid, giddy. They come under different headings, and different brand names, and then the brand names vary from country to country. Knowing something about the different types should make it a little less bewildering once you actually go into labour and hear all those words being bandied about.

Analgesia is the general term for drugs which relieve pain without necessarily inducing sleep. Hypnotics are given usually during the early part of labour and are specifically to induce sleep but do not in themselves directly relieve pain. Sedatives relieve anxiety and produce a feeling of calm or drowsiness without necessarily inducing sleep, although when given in strong doses they do make you sleepy, so they then have to be classed as hypnotics. Tranquillizers are also not directly pain-relievers but are designed to relieve anxiety and tension; again, in larger doses they do make you want to sleep. Anaesthesia obviously relieves pain as it blots out all sensation, either by inducing unconsciousness, as in a general anaesthetic, or by temporarily blocking the routes by which sensory nerves communicate pain sensations to the brain, as in a 'local' or 'conduction' anaesthetic.

It is easier to make the decision as to whether you use drugs during labour, if you know beforehand the possible effects of anaesthetics, analgesics and sedatives on mother and child.

Before the mid-nineteenth century, it seems women managed without much medicinal relief, and after that opium and its derivatives became the main source of comfort. A mixture of morphine and scopolamine, the first an especially strong analgesic, termed a narcotic, the second an hypnotic which induces sleep and makes your mouth dry, was introduced in Germany in 1907. It was called 'twilight sleep' because it put the woman into a state somewhere between consciousness and unconsciousness. Injections of heroin, supplemented by nitrous oxide gas given through a face mask, were the next step in labour pain relief. Heroin and morphine are both analgesics and derivatives of opium. Nitrous oxide, or laughing gas, is an inhalant anaesthetic, usually only used in the final stages of delivery.

Today's most popular drug for labour is Pethidine in England, called Meperidine in the U.S.A. (the proprietary name is Demerol)—strong, and a synthetic substitute for morphine and heroin. Often given with scopolamine, the drugs not only numb sensation but also erase the memory of it. Pethidine, combined with Levallorphan, which is used to combat the nauseous side-effects, becomes Pethilorfan. In England Sparine is frequently added to Pethidine to counteract the nauseous side-effects of the first, and reinforce its action. Sparine itself makes you sleepy, and in combination with such a heavy analgesic as Pethidine, can keep you completely out of the action, too far out of it to stay in touch with the rhythm of strong contractions. Barbiturates, which are sleeping pills (i.e. Seconal), have much the same effect, and, being profound sedatives, can cause a pronounced fall in a woman's blood pressure. They slow you down which is why they are called 'downers' in the idiom of those who take them regularly. Since they cross the placenta, they have the same depressant effect on the baby.

Analgesics can be given orally or by hypodermic injection directly into a vein or muscle. Intravenous injections work the most rapidly. The drug goes straight into the bloodstream and immediately affects the brain, making reality seem fuzzy and distant.

Epidurals and Caudal blocks, anaesthetics injected around the spinal nerves, leaving the mental consciousness of the mother unclouded, were originally developed for clinical surgery. Such anaesthesia provides a fairly easy answer to dulling the sensation of contractions. It is estimated that epidurals are now being used in about 2 per cent of the 800,000 deliveries a year in Britain. One setback is that the absolute lack of sensation, which it causes in about 50 per cent of women, takes away the woman's urge to push and utilize contractions to help in the delivery of her baby. Moreover, the epidural usually weakens the muscles used in pushing, so leading to more and more forceps deliveries.

Effects of Labour Drugs on the Baby

If we, as grown women, are susceptible to powerful painkilling and sedating drugs, it is obvious that since they cross the placenta, the baby within us, just a fraction of our size, is likely to feel the effects more seriously. A heavy dose of an analgesic, strong enough to relieve labour pains effectively in a mother, and possibly knock her out, or make her very very sleepy, will also make the baby sleepy. The woman has a lowering of blood pressure and depression of respiration, which means her breathing becomes less efficient; this will affect the baby's breathing, if he is delivered within two or three hours of the dose being administered.[1] The normal dose for Pethidine, for instance, is 100 mg; 200 mg would have a very strong effect. Since it is considered quite normal to give more than one 100 mg dose during a labour, if you really want something it is sensible to ask for 50 mg and see if it helps you enough to leave it at that. Mild or strong, it will reach the baby.

Dr Yvonne Brackbill, Professor of Obstetrics, Gynaecology and Paediatrics for Psychology at Georgetown University, has said that Pethidine (Meperidine) is used in 80 to 90 per cent of all deliveries in Great Britain.[2] Her study of mother—infant interaction provided clear evidence that 'Meperidine produces outstanding neo-natal differences in ability to process information', and that to her 'a major obstetric danger may now be medication itself'.

1. *Pregnancy* by Gordon Bourne, F.R.C.S., F.R.C.O.G., p. 360, London, 1972.
2. *American Journal of Obstetrics and Gynecology*, 1st February, 1974.

Knowing that the placenta is not a barrier, as was once thought, but more like a sieve, through which all chemicals pass to the child, the responsibility for the drugs we take with a child inside us is in our hands.

'The respiratory center of the infant is highly susceptible to sedative and anaesthetic drugs administered to the mother',[1] say the American doctors Hellman and Pritchard, researching the after-effects of drugs on the newborn. They found infants born to a sedated mother 'sluggish', and feel this could jeopardize the efficiency of their respiration in the crucial first moments of life.

In 1970, the Society for Research in Child Development published a report,[2] which was summarized in the International Childbirth Education Association:[3]

'Virtually all obstetric medications—nausea remedies, diuretics, sedatives, muscle relaxants, analgesics, regional anaesthesia and general anaesthetics—tend to rapidly cross the placenta and alter the fetal environment as they enter the circulatory system of the unborn infant within seconds or minutes of administration to the mother.'

A drug which stays in the mother's bloodstream two hours could take two days for the baby to eliminate. Dr Robert A. Bradley, M.D., obstetrician and author,[4] says of drugs given during labour:

'The mother weighs 140 pounds, while the baby weighs seven; yet they both get the same dosage (of drugs). So if you give the mother an adequate dose, enough to put her out, you are giving the baby twenty times as heavy a dose.'

Sedatives containing barbiturates and strong analgesics such as Pethidine (Meperidine) affect a child's sucking reflexes, and drugs given during labour can cut down the possibility of nursing. They

1. Hellman, L. and Pritchard, J.: *Williams Obstetrics*, 14th edition, New York, 1971.

2. Bowes *et al.*: 'The Effects of Obstetrical Medication on Fetus and Infant', monograph of the Society for Research in Child Development, No. 137, Volume 35, June 1970, U.S.A.

3. *The Cultural Warping of Childbirth*, a special report by Doris Haine, co-President, International Childbirth Education Association, p. 10, 1972, U.S.A.

4. *Husband-Coached Childbirth*, New York: Harper & Row.

make infants sleepy and unresponsive.[1] One study shows a twenty-four-hour delay in the baby's weight gain, delayed sucking response, and abnormalities during the early days after birth.[2]

Local, or regional, anaesthetics such as the epidural (or extradural) are thought of by most people as relatively harmless to mother and child. However, research shows they too can threaten the health of unborn and newly born babies.[3] In a group of ninety-three mothers studied in America after receiving paracervical block anaesthesia,[4] there was a temporary drop in the babies' heart rate in almost half the group. In another series studied by the same doctors, infant depression of heart rate, respiration and muscle-tone was almost three times greater in those whose mothers had received this anaesthesia than in those who had not. An abnormal drop in a child's heart rate usually indicates a decrease in his oxygen supply. One of the great difficulties of this kind of obstetric medication is that nobody really knows how much loss of oxygen can be sustained by a child in labour or just after birth, before there is neurological damage. Even minimal brain damage can affect a child's personality and his ability to learn.

In human beings, the peak in the velocity curve of brain growth occurs around the time of birth. In other animals, this peak rate will come either before birth, as with guinea-pigs, or afterwards, as in rats.[5] This, coupled with the inherent dangers of asphyxia (suffocation), anoxia (lack of oxygen), and vulnerability of the central nervous system (that part of us most affected by drugs), probably means human babies are uniquely susceptible to brain damage at

1. Richards, M. P. M.: *Feeding and Early Growth of the Mother-Child Relationship*, pp. 13–14, published by Karger, Basel, 1973.

2. Constance Bean, 'Methods of Childbirth', study by Dr T. Brazelton, 1968. Johnson, W.: 'Regionals can Prolong Labor', *Medical World News*, 15th October, 1971.

3. Vasicky, A.: 'Foetal Bradycardis after Paracervical Block', *Obstetrics and Gynecology*, 38: 500, 1971 (U.S.A.). Johnson, W.: 'Regionals can Prolong Labor', *Medical World News*, 15th October, 1971.

4. Rosefsky, J. and Petersiel, M.: 'Perinatal Deaths Associated with Mepivacaine Paracervical Block Anesthesia in Labor', *New England Journal of Medicine*, 278: 530, 1968.

5. Richards, Dr Martin: 'An Ecological Study of Infant Development in an Urban Setting in Britain', ed. Leiderman, Tulkin, February 1974, published by Stamford University Press.

birth. Just knowing this single fact makes a difference to the attention we should pay to the quality of care we give our children at delivery.

There seems little doubt that analgesics given in large doses during labour may indirectly have a lasting effect on the relationship between a woman and her newborn child. Analgesics are nervous depressants, depressing not only pain but all sensation and other nervous mechanisms including emotional responses. The babies suffer from respiratory depression, are slower to breathe and cry at birth, and slower to develop the sucking reflex. Dr Martin Richards, lecturer in social psychology at the Unit for Research on the Medical Applications of Psychology in Cambridge, England, has been studying the relationships between mothers and children from birth to school age, and finds that there is a marked difference in behaviour if the labour is drugged.

His work[1] shows there is also a clear connection between drugs, usually Pethilorfan, given during labour and the feeling of separation between mothers and infants after birth. He says that:

'The clearest case of psychological separation occurs when the mothers receive an analgesic drug during labour . . . After the administration of Pethilorfan, infants suffer from mild respiratory depression and are slower to cry and breathe at birth.'[2]

He found that the length of the babies' feeds are shorter after Pethilorfan, the babies are sleepy and unresponsive, and mothers have to work to get them to stay awake and suck. At both thirty and sixty weeks babies and mothers have less intimate contact, and babies show more 'self-stimulatory' activities, like thumb-sucking. He points out that although they as yet have no definite information beyond the first year:

'It is unlikely that an event that has led to a different path of development in the first twelve months will not continue to have some influence.'

1. Richards, Dr Martin: 'An Ecological Study of Infant Development in an Urban Setting in Britain', ed. Liederman, Tulkin, February 1974, published by Stamford University Press.
2. Richards, Dr Martin: 'One Day Old Deprived Child', p. 820, *New Scientist*, 28th March, 1974.

The observations are summed up by reiterating how cautious we should be about dismissing drug effects as trivial before we know absolutely that they are so.

Dr J. Aidan McFarlane, M.R.C.P., researching and evaluating the effects of obstetric procedures on mother-child interaction, at the obstetric unit of the John Radcliffe Hospital, Oxford, England, has found that his own work substantiates the conclusions reached by various other investigators in this field. Obstetric medication given to the mother affects the infant in a number of ways. This includes sucking, attention, muscle tension, and orientation.[1]

He told me that he finds a notable lowering of the baby's pulse rate, respiratory rate, heart rate, oxygen level in the blood, and sucking reflex, if the woman has been given drugs in labour. Many women believe children cannot see at birth, but he maintains that not only do they see, but the degree to which they focus can be altered by the amount of medication a mother has had. He finds that women who have not been heavily sedated want to handle their babies immediately after birth, have instant skin contact, naked if possible, so that there is a build-up of warmth between the two right away, have eye-to-eye contact from the early moments and touch their babies with their fingertips and the palms of their hands particularly.[2]

It is obviously difficult to test labour drugs exhaustively on human mothers or infants, as few women would be prepared to be guinea-pigs while giving birth, yet in fact most women are. There is no way of testing the effects of these drugs as they cross the placenta and reach the baby, before they are put into general use. They may trigger off any number of hormonal changes, the type and results of which can only be recorded through clinical observation of the fact—or by listening to the feelings of the women who are giving birth.

As Professor Davis, paediatric specialist at St Mary's Hospital, Manchester, stated on B.B.C. television, during a programme examining the pros and cons of induction[3]:

1. Kron *et al.*: 'Newborn Sucking Behaviour Affected by Obstetric Sedation', *Pediatrics*, 37: 1012, 1966.
Stechler: 'Newborn Attention as Affected by Medication during Labour', *Science*, 144: 315, 1964
Brackbill: 'The Effects of Obstetrical Medication on Foetus and Infant', monographs of the Society for Research in Child Development, 35: No. 4, 1970.
2. See also Marshal Klaus, M.D., 'Maternal Attachment—Importance of the First Post-Partum Days', *New England Journal of Medicine*, March 1972.
3. B.B.C.2, *Horizon*, 'A Time to be Born', 27th January, 1975.

'The onus is on the medical profession to prove that a pharmacological labour is superior.'

In other words, it is not up to us to prove that what now seems to
be excessive use of medication is wrong, but rather up to those who
have created these conditions to prove they are right. And this has
not yet been done. He also points to the increase in neonatal jaundice,
enlargement of spleen, floppiness of muscles and the need for
resuscitation, where a birth has been artificially induced, heavily
sedated because of the suddenness of the onset of pain in an induced
labour, with most probably an epidural anaesthetic and forceps
delivery. He is honest enough to admit that these results worry him
because, he says, 'I don't know why they happen'.

Babies die more frequently from causes relative to the amount of
medication given to the mother in the United States than in any
other country. Drugs are widely used during pregnancy, labour and
delivery, in America, and a survey taken of thirteen countries in
1972 shows America as having the highest infant mortality rate
(5·5 in every 1,000 live births)[1] due to post-natal asphyxia and birth
injuries—conditions 'which are more likely to occur if the mother
has received obstetrical medication'.[2]

1. *Infant Mortality Rates (per 1,000 Live Births) in Selected Countries*

	all causes	birth injuries, post-natal asphyxia and atelectasis
	%	%
Canada	22·0	4·5
U.S.A.	22·4	5·5
Japan	14·9	1·7
Belgium	22·9	3·0
Denmark	15·8	5·3
Finland	14·8	5·4
Norway	14·8	4·2
Netherlands	13·4	3·6
England and Wales	18·3	4·5
Sweden	12·9	4·3
Switzerland	17·5	4·4
New Zealand	18·0	4·6

Information based on statistics available from Statistical Office of the United
Nations, taken in 1967, published in the I.C.E.A. Special Report on *The Cultural
Warping of Childbirth*, 1972.

2. Quote from I.C.E.A. News Special Report on *The Cultural Warping of
Childbirth*, by the co-President of the International Childbirth Education
Association, Mrs Doris Haire, p. 8, published 1972.

These figures are based on United Nations statistics, and the report is a result of the experience of Mrs Doris Haire, co-President of America's International Childbirth Education Association. Mrs Haire claims that in her world travels, gathering information on birth conditions and techniques, she has found the mortality rate figures relate to a difference in cultural attitude towards birth, and babies die less frequently in countries where midwives form an essential part of obstetrical care, both in and out of hospital; where the physician is only called in when the pregnant woman is ill or the birth is expected to be in some way abnormal; and where mothers are actively encouraged to breastfeed their children. Her grim conclusion is that if statistics follow the present trend, a child born in the United States is four times more likely to die in the first day of life than an infant born, say, in Japan.

In the light of this kind of information, a woman's request to have her baby naturally, if she so wishes, becomes rather more serious than simply an emotional plea—it is a challenge to all of us to consider whether excessive and undiscriminating recourse to technology might in fact be endangering the lives of our children.

Labour Drug Terminology

The following lists are of the general categories of drugs you are most likely to encounter during labour, and then those specific drugs widely used in birth procedures. All medication crosses the placenta and affects the fetal environment. The extent to which it happens is dependent on the amount of the drug you take, and whether or not it has an analgesic or anaesthetic effect upon you. In other words, the more strongly you are affected, the more strongly your changes will be absorbed through the placenta and picked up by the baby. The route of administration of drugs affects the rate at which they cross the placenta. A rough estimate is: by mouth, 2 to 4 hours; by intra-muscular injection, 30 to 120 minutes; by intra-venous injection, 2 to 30 minutes.

GENERAL TERMS

Analgesic: general term to describe a drug which relieves pain without necessarily inducing sleep, although it may do so.

anaesthetic (general)	leads to total loss of consciousness; the reflex action is abolished; depression of motor centres followed by depression of muscular tone, pulse and respiration.
anaesthetic (local or conduction)	affects a limited region of the body obliterating sensation in that area only.
narcotic	produces abnormally deep sleep as well as having pain-relieving properties; quickly causes dependence and is fatal in overdose; may be of organic origin (i.e. morphine and codeine) or derivative of the organic substance (heroin), or synthetic, producing the same effect (Pethidine/Meperidine).
Sedatives:	general term to describe drugs which relieve anxiety and possibly make you feel drowsy, with no specific effect on pain.
tranquillizers	these are used to relieve anxiety and promote calmness without inducing sleep or lessening pain.
barbiturates	are used in small doses as a sedative to relieve anxiety and in larger doses as a sleeping pill. Slow-acting barbiturates have no effect on pain, and so compounds with analgesics have been devised. The hypnotic action is largely responsible for some decrease in the blood pressure, pulse rate and bowel activity. Heavy doses lower the blood pressure considerably.
hypnotics	lead to depression of the sensory functions of the brain and the reflex activity of the spinal cord. They are usually given in the early stages of labour. The effects are sleepiness, impaired co-ordination, then depression of reflexes while maintaining consciousness, and without affecting the

sensation of pain. Considerably stronger doses can lead to complete loss of consciousness.

TYPES OF LABOUR DRUGS

Analgesics: for the relief of pain, these can be administered either orally, by injection into the muscles or the veins.

Pethidine/Meperidine U.K. U.S.A. (trade name in U.S.A. is *Demerol*) synthetic narcotic analgesic, usually injected during the first stage of labour in regulated doses; it takes away the sharp edge of pain and has a slightly hypnotic effect; you could doze in between contractions; this drug is given almost everywhere now in place of heroin or morphine, which used to be the most widely administered labour analgesics; supposedly Pethidine cuts out their side-effects of nausea and dizziness, but some people find themselves still affected adversely.

Pethilorfan this is Pethidine plus its narcotic antagonist, Levallorphan, administered at the same stages and in the same way as Pethidine to reduce the nauseous side-effects of Pethidine.

Morphine powerful pain-relieving narcotic which also induces sleep in anything but the smallest doses; derived from opium; usually administered intravenously; it is also an euphoriant which means it has the quality of making you feel peculiarly cheerful.

Scopolamine used to be given in combination with Morphine to create 'twilight sleep'; it can cause hallucinations and dry the mucous secretions in nose and throat.

79

Sparine

this is a tranquillizer (Promazine) and like Phenergan (Promethazine) is more often given in combination with something like Pethidine, than alone; this is because both drugs have the effect of reducing anxiety and tension as well as controlling or reducing nausea and vomiting—very often the side-effects of the stronger, narcotic, analgesics.

Inhalant analgesics:

usually administered in the final stages of labour by means of a mask held over the mouth, either by an anaesthetist or the woman herself; analgesia starts about 20 seconds after first inhalation; these types of analgesia or anaesthetics cross the placenta, as do drugs given orally or intravenously, and affect the baby, particularly when they follow other pain-relieving drugs such as Pethidine; this makes the baby very sleepy, so causing breathing difficulties after delivery because of reduced oxygen intake to the brain and tissues.

Nitrous oxide

known as 'laughing gas'; it causes a rushing noise in the ears, blurred vision, giddiness, euphoria, and hilarity if the amount inhaled is too low to produce unconsciousness; respiration becomes difficult if inhalation lasts longer than 30 seconds, and there may be signs of asphyxia; it does possess a relatively strong pain-relieving action which can have the side-effect of nausea; the gas has a depressant effect on the nervous system and respiratory centre, but no direct influence on the heart.

Entonox

a mixture of 50 per cent nitrous oxide and 50 per cent oxygen, introduced because nitrous oxide alone has such a depressant effect on both mother and child; this combination is mixed before use in a cylinder and the increased level of oxygen present in the analgesic benefits both mother and child, in comparison to the effect of pure nitrous oxide; Entonox does not cause loss of consciousness, nor does it have side-effects, although its efficacy as a pain-reliever is not so total as with nitrous oxide alone.

Trilene essentially similar to nitrous oxide and Entonox, this can be used as an anaesthetic in concentrated dose; when it causes rapid loss of consciousness and moderate muscular relaxation there is a build-up of analgesia after you have inhaled with the first few contractions, because it is not exhaled immediately from the lungs, so the elimination of Trilene from a mother's blood and tissues is comparatively slow; the safe dosage is 0·5 per cent or less of Trilene vapour in air.

Local analgesia: an injection which blocks the nerves that supply sensation to a specific part of the body, without causing unconsciousness.

For an episiotomy the perineum is injected with local anaesthetic which works almost at once so the episiotomy can be performed quickly and painlessly.

Pudendal nerve block a type of regional anaesthesia administered just before a forceps delivery. The pudendal nerves supply sensation to most of the perineum, the vulva, the vagina, and the muscles of the pelvic floor. The nerves in the side wall of the pelvis are injected with local anaesthetic, so numbing that area completely.

Paracervical block: this is most effective during the first stage of labour, and can only be performed when the cervix is less than 5 centimetres in diameter. It blocks sensation for between three to four hours, and is injected into the plexus, where most of the nerves that supply the uterus and cervix are collected. Thus the uterus becomes completely insensitive.

Conduction anaesthetics: a cocaine drug such as Xylocaine or Novocaine is injected at a specific location to block nerve impulses to the brain. A skilled anaesthetist is essential. The woman remains conscious. She can usually move her legs but the urge to bear down is inhibited.

Epidural: in the usual kind of epidurals (lumbar block), an injection of anaesthetic which numbs the lower abdomen and legs, usually down to the feet, is administered during labour. It is given into the epidural cavity—the space lined by ligament and bone, external to the dura, that tough membrane which covers the spinal cord. With an epidural there is no contact with the spinal cord itself. For a continuous epidural, a soft catheter is introduced through a needle into the epidural space, and the anaesthetic can then be given over a prolonged period of time. Such analgesia is generally thought to be very effective to relieve a mother's pain from contractions. However, it does cross the placenta and alters the fetal environment and it does mean that the absolute lack of sensation, which it causes in about 50 per cent of women, takes away the urge to push and utilize contractions to help in the delivery of the baby, with the possible result of a lengthy labour necessitating a forceps delivery. It is essential to keep checking blood pressure, strength of contractions and signs of the progression of labour such as dilation of the cervix and position of the baby in the birth canal, as the woman will be unable to feel any of this naturally.

Caudal block : this is administered by an injection in the lowest, sacral, region of the spine and affects only the lower pelvic area. Effects on the mother, the progression of labour and the baby are likely to be similar to the epidural. The difference between the two technically is that an epidural anaesthetic is injected into the lumbar region of the spine, and the caudal goes into the tip of the spine in the region of the coccyx.

Spinal anaesthesia : this is the single injection of a local anaesthetic solution into the tissue space which immediately surrounds the spinal cord, and can be given only once during labour. It lasts for about two hours. Controversy mystifies the efficiency of this method, because although it definitely eliminates pain for the mother, it has had serious side-effects. Some women have excruciating headaches, lasting for some days after delivery, and there are rumours of serious dangers to mother and child should it be used improperly. This may be why it is not popular, or used very often, in either Europe or America today.

PROS AND CONS OF CONDUCTION ANAESTHETICS

Valid medical reasons: if the mother has high blood pressure, because epidurals tend to lower the blood pressure;

83

cardiac or respiratory distress in the mother during labour;

heart disease;

an obstetric abnormality which might make labour more difficult to handle for some women. This would be if the baby was in an abnormal position in the womb, which can cause acute labour discomfort not normally controlled by the standard labour analgesics.

Hazardous side effects: a dural puncture if the anaesthetic is administered inefficiently, or the mother should move inadvertently during administration, with resulting severe headache for which the only cure is to lie flat on your back in bed for some time after delivery;

supine hypotension (low blood pressure) resulting from anaesthesia in the spine;

possible nerve damage or even infection if carelessly administered;

the anaesthetic affects the bladder so there may be difficulty in passing water during the post-delivery period;

can cause faintness and nausea;

there is a risk of paralysis.

Reasons specifically to avoid: if you have any vaginal bleeding during pregnancy or early labour;

lack of adequate facilities for its administration where you are having your baby since it is a highly complex and delicate procedure requiring expert knowledge and experience;

if the mother has certain neurological conditions (check with your doctor);

supine hypotension, which is a pronounced fall in blood pressure; as conduction anaesthetics lower the maternal blood pressure in any case, it would be unwise for a woman with this low blood pressure condition to have such an anaesthetic.

Mechanical Intervention in Labour

INDUCTION

Induction is the method of artificially stimulating the uterus into labour contractions, with the intention of controlling the birth of a baby.

Quinine was the first drug used for inductions. Now the most usual artificial stimulant is the synthetic analogue of a natural hormone, oxytocin. This is the hormone generated by the mother's pituitary gland in natural labour to make the uterus contract. Its synthetic analogue has the same effect on the uterus. However, dosage of the synthetic hormone is crucial and one has to allow for the risk of human error. Other uterine stimulants, prostaglandins, appear to have the same effects: they not only induce, or trigger off, labour, but also intensify the frequency and strength of contractions.

Induction usually begins when the membranes are ruptured; then a catheter is fitted to the arm of the mother so as to maintain a constant drip of the induction agent into her vein. Once attached to this contraption, a woman cannot change her mind and come off it, as such a move would increase the danger of hemorrhage.

Although induction for social or medical convenience is quite a new turn of events, inductions themselves have been used by obstetricians for many years in cases where there was clear-cut doubt as to the health of either the mother or the baby if the baby were allowed to remain in the womb. For instance if the mother had diabetes, toxemia, there was danger of hemorrhage, or the pregnancy was going over time. Prolonged pregnancy becomes a danger to the baby when it goes more than fourteen days beyond the expected date of delivery, because there is a possibility the placenta will cease to nourish the baby adequately.

Having been introduced for very good reason, induction for social convenience is now being encouraged by some gynaecologists, and a number of hospitals have tried to bring in a policy of 'nine to five deliveries' because they fear that shortage of night staff might endanger the night-born babies. However, according to the English medical paper, *The Lancet*, there is some evidence to suggest that babies born during the day might be more 'vulnerable to the kind of distress that requires oxygen administration'.[1]

In some obstetric units in England, half, or more, of the women are not permitted to go into spontaneous labour, usually because inductions are the general policy of the hospitals they attend. Supposedly, hospitals find it easier to control labour by pharmacological means (drugs) than to encourage women to manage their own labours. Yet this is despite the fact that the timing of delivery is naturally controlled by complex mechanisms within us that are only barely understood by man, but which have as their ultimate goal the safe delivery of a child.[2]

The chief dangers of using uterine stimulants are to the baby. Errors in judgement are bound to happen in any large group of elective inductions. There is no woman I know who is ever completely certain of her dates, and very few who always have completely regular menstrual cycles—so there is probably no way of being 100 per cent correct in judging whether a baby has gone 'full term' or not, and induction may mean a very real possibility of premature birth.

'There will inevitably be a proportion of cases in which an error in dating of gestation results in a premature child who may die or suffer irreparable damage in the neonatal period.'

So says *The Lancet*.[3] Obviously there are inherent dangers to induction, in addition to which it is possible that some children need more time than others in the womb—for many different reasons, from the mental and physical state of the mother to the environmental conditions of pregnancy.

There seems to be a definite relationship between oxytocin being used to induce labour, abnormally strong contractions and fetal heart distress.[4] Reports linking fetal problems with excessively

1. 'A Time to be Born', p. 1183, *The Lancet*, 16th November, 1974.
2. Klopper, A., Gardner, J. (editors), *Endocrine Factors in Labour*, London, 1973.
3. *The Lancet*, p. 1183, 16th November, 1974.
4. Professor Davis, Queen Mary's Hospital, Manchester, speaking on B.B.C.2 television, *Horizon*, 27th January, 1975.

frequent contractions usually reflect misuse of the drug. High doses of oxytocin can lead to fetal morbidity during labour and after delivery.[1]

According to research in Cardiff and Oxford, and the experience of Professor Davis, paediatric specialist at Queen Mary's Hospital, Manchester, there is an increase in babies with jaundice which relates directly to artificial induction. In its most severe form, jaundice could lead to a degree of brain damage, although as a rule it is fairly mild. Professor Davis has also found a tendency to use more sedative medicines in induced delivery because of the increase in discomfort from abnormally strong and frequent contractions.

In the United States, research by the doctors Hellman and Pritchard[2] has led them to caution that the conveniences of elective induction are not without 'the attendant hazards of prematurity, prolonged latent period with intrapartum infection, and prolapse of the umbilical cord'.

They report that studies involving almost 10,000 elective inductions indicate that perinatal deaths due to inductions administered too soon, when the baby is very premature, still happen even though obstetricians try their best to comply with specific medical criteria.

Also in the States, after studying 3,324 inductions at the University of Pennsylvania, H. Fields, who recorded the result,[3] has this to say:

'The hazards of the use of oxytocin in labor are related directly to the dose for the given individual. Overdosage results in uterine spasms with possible separation of the placenta, tumultuous labor, amniotic fluid embolus, afibrinogenemia, lacerations of the cervix and birth canal, postpartum hemorrhage and uterine rupture. There may be water intoxication due to the antidiuretic effect of oxytocin. There may be fetal distress due to anoxia and intracranial hemorrhage, and trauma may result from tumultuous uterine contractions. Fetal and/or maternal mortality are, of course, ever present dangers.'

1. Gosh, A., Hudson, F. P., *The Lancet*, p. 823, 1972.
2. Hellman, L., Pritchard, J.: *Williams Obstetrics*, 14th edition, New York, 1971.
3. Field, H.: 'Complications of Elective Inductions', *Obstetrics and Gynecology*, 15: 476, 1960.

Meaning that if anyone were to slip up and give you a bit too much, things might get pretty unpleasant.

Any kind of anaesthetics can, like alcohol, leave almighty hangovers. Anaesthetics or analgesics are commonly used during an induced labour, so are forceps. One artificial intervention tends to lead to another, so that drugs which induce labour often bring on contractions of such force that more painkillers are used, rendering the woman less able to manage her own labour, probably less able to push and so deliver her child without the help of forceps.

Although it is too soon to judge the long-term effects of artificially starting and controlling a normal labour, it is now thought that in a natural labour the fetus itself might play a key part in initiating contractions, as well as preparing the lungs for breathing.[1] The baby receives less oxygen during a contraction, so tumultuous contractions could lead to further and unnecessary oxygen deprivation.

The gradual build-up in intensity of natural labour, which starts spontaneously and goes on without chemical stimulation, allows a woman time to adjust to the pace of her labour, perhaps even develop some tolerance to its discomforts. This may well be a natural protective mechanism for both mother and baby that whenever possible is best left untampered with.

To me the most relevant point for women who know that their babies are perfectly healthy and showing no signs of distress, is that hormone drips and inductions do tend to make labour 'tumultuous'. In such a case preparation will help, but however well prepared, you could find it very difficult to handle artificially paced contractions.

Make sure to check with your doctor *why* he is recommending induction.

Valid reasons:	if you have high blood pressure, or any indications of toxemia;
	diabetes;
	when the baby is smaller than expected, or more than fourteen days over expected date of delivery;
	small maternal pelvis.

1. Dawes, G. S.: 'Hazards of Birth', p. 135, *Human Reproduction: from the Science Journal*, London, 1971.

Dangers:	small or premature babies, when induced, have a higher risk of dying after they are born, because they cannot use their lungs sufficiently.
Inconveniences:	tougher labour, although shorter, strengthens and speeds up contractions, making them more difficult to deal with; can lead to hospital administering an epidural anaesthetic, if they think the mother is too tired to cope with extra pressures of discomfort and increased pain, which in turn could lead to a forceps delivery.

CAESAREAN

The Caesarean section is basically the delivery of a baby via an incision in the womb, rather than through the normal passage from cervix to vagina. It is a major operation, requiring a general anaesthetic, and you are unlikely to know anything about it until you wake up in bed.

A Caesarean is indicated when there are 'mechanical' difficulties in the way of a normal birth, a woman has had a Caesarean delivery before, or for reasons which might make normal delivery very difficult.

There are two kinds of incision used for Caesarean delivery—one longitudinal from a point below the navel to a point above the cervix, the other transverse, usually low down on the edge of or below the pubic hair line. The latter is known as 'the bikini cut'. Of the two types of incision, most women, if they know they have a choice, opt for the latter, which is often scarcely visible once the hair has grown back.

FORCEPS

These are large spoon-like implements which were originally used when the baby was literally in a very tight situation, and had already suffered harm, so that the instrument came to be associated with 'damaged' babies. Forceps used in particularly difficult deliveries are usually termed 'high forceps' because they reach further up the birth canal.

Today a baby is seldom delivered with forceps unless it is already two-thirds of the way through the birth canal ('low forceps'). Forceps are sometimes used to turn the baby into a more favourable position before gently pulling him out, but mostly they are used as a shoe-horn, to ease the baby out. They are always applied round the baby's head.

The use of forceps is particularly relevant if the baby is premature, or expected to be small, or is in a breech position (bottom first). The increasing use of anaesthetics and strong analgesics also implies a higher forceps delivery rate—a woman who has had epidural anaesthesia, for example, has an inhibited desire to push, because she experiences so little feeling.

EPISIOTOMY

This is the long word for a small surgical incision performed with scissors during labour. A cut is made in the skin between vagina and anus, the perineum, especially when forceps are used.

A doctor will do this if he feels labour is being delayed by the skin of the perineum not 'giving' enough; or if he thinks your skin will tear when the baby's head comes through, he will cut the skin himself. On the other hand you might not tear at all. You do not feel either a tear or a cut very much because when the perineum begins to stretch you do not know whether you are burning or freezing—nature works its own anaesthetic.

If you do have one, ask about a local anaesthetic before stitching up after delivery. Internal stitches usually take some days to dissolve, and there is unlikely to be any alteration to the size of your vagina. If you have skin stitches, they will have to be removed separately.

CARDIOGRAPH

The cardiograph, phonocardiograph and electrocardiograph are three machines used to monitor the course of labour and the baby's condition. Their use is becoming standard procedure in many large hospitals.

The electrocardiograph employs electrodes attached to the baby's scalp or mother's abdomen, which record his condition on a paper print-out closely watched for any abnormality.

The cardiograph uses ultrasound for the same purpose.

The phonocardiograph uses a special microphone to allow doctors to hear the fetal heartbeat.

In the United States there is now one machine instead of three, and this one machine does all the work described above. It is called a 'fetal monitor'.

THE CARDIFF INFUSION UNIT: MACHINE-CONTROLLED LABOUR

This baby machine manages to combine just about everything needed for an artificial labour. The woman has a strap round her stomach attached to a machine, which then automatically induces, monitors, controls and helps to deliver the baby by dilating the cervix.

The induction agents used in computer-controlled labour are oxytocin and prostaglandins. Both, it is now known, cause a rise of bile pigment level in the baby's blood.[1] The machine can also 'administer' Pethidine as a painkiller. If contractions become unbearably strong because of the induction, it will then regulate their intensity by altering the rate at which the stimulating hormone is dripped to the mother intravenously. The contractions are monitored by way of a catheter threaded into the vagina, through the birth canal and inserted into the neck of the womb.

The woman must stay on the machine for at least thirty minutes after delivery as the strong inducing hormones increase risk of maternal hemorrhage.

It is said by doctors to be giving women an advantage to have a strap around their abdomens so they can watch the length and strength of contractions on the dials of their computer. However, a strap round your abdomen during labour can be very unpleasant. The skin during labour is particularly sensitive to touch and this kind of restriction could make a woman reluctant to get off her back. It is not only a psychological disadvantage to be on one's back while trying to deal with contractions through breathing patterns and conscious relaxation, it is also extremely uncomfortable.

1. *The Lancet*, p. 1339, 7th December, 1974.

4

The Re-Humanization of Birth

'*There is no greater joy than that of a woman who sees her baby born, hears its greeting and holds it in her hands whilst it is still linked to her body by the avenue through which its life-blood surged from the selective source within her womb.*'

Childbirth Without Fear, GRANTLY DICK-READ

Don't Cut the Cord too Soon: Dr R. D. Laing

Dr Laing is a psychiatrist, author and father of eight, much concerned with the effect of modern obstetrical practice on the psyche of our children. He believes that experiences at birth and in the womb have reverberations on our mental state for the rest of our lives. He believes the nervous system of a baby is sufficiently developed at the time of being born to store up memories which echo into later life and lead to disturbance. From the earliest stages of gestation, each individual is affected by whether or not it is wanted, and the way in which it is welcomed into our world. By cutting the umbilical cord too quickly he feels a baby may be put into a state of extreme, and unnecessary, shock.

In October, 1972 he drew the attention of psychiatrists, paediatricians and gynaecologists to his views when he spoke at the inaugural meeting of the British section of the International Society of Psychosomatic Obstetrics and Gynaecology.[1] In a discussion on

1. The Inaugural Meeting of the British Section of the I.S.P.O.G. took place at the Royal Society of Medicine, London, on 28th October, 1972. Quotations here are taken from tapes made at the time.

'The Family—Present and Future', Dr Laing found leading obstetricians openly agreeing with his admonition that those in charge of delivering our children be more aware of and responsible for a baby's extreme sensitivity at the moment of birth.

Dr Laing opened his talk by saying that he had been browsing among obstetric textbooks, and found absolutely no reference to the fact that a baby actually experiences being born. He admitted that when he was a medical student it had not occurred to him that a baby might have feelings, or if it had, then he dismissed it because his neuro-physiological dogma was that experience is not yet being recorded at the time of birth. Since then he has changed his mind. He has begun to remember his own birth.

'I don't think behavioural studies will settle the matter of whether or not we feel as we are being born. I think it comes down to one's own memory. Before I felt I could remember any of my own birth, I was influenced by the sermon of the Buddha, in which the first Noble Truth he presents to us, independent of time, place, socio-economic and cultural circumstances, is that birth, old age, illness and death are painful. I think there's no doubt that he actually meant that when we're born, we experience it.

'I spend a lot of my time meeting all sorts of people, and among them are people who have very clear early memories, a definite record of their early input and central processing. They say they can remember their birth better than their first visit to the seaside. I think most people don't remember anything about it because it was so overwhelmingly felt that some switch was shut off and it was repressed.'

His observation of humanity is that many of us partially remember our births, and enact this first remembered scenario over and over again during adult life.

'Some people never get over it,' he said. 'They spend their lives staggering around under the repeated impulses of stored and activated impressions. They are registered somewhere in the baby's organism and later reproduce themselves as muscle tension, body tics, all sorts of anxieties which affect cardiac rhythms, breathing function and may underlie otherwise inexplicable allergies, upper respiratory tract infections, asthma, and phobias of being in an enclosed space.

'It's an abstract dynamic geometry, an experience of being in something that in the first place one doesn't want to be in, which is coming in on one from all sides. There seems to be no way out of it, no way to avoid or evade it. It is out of one's control and beyond one's capacity to endure. The feeling is that one is at an *impasse*. One is being oppressed or compressed, possibly even crushed and ground down, finished, reducing one to a sense of complete impotence where all one's resources have failed, and there's nothing more one can do.

'Then, just when it seems to be utterly hopeless, something begins to happen. It may not be something better, but at least there is a change taking place, and, through what may be many adventures, some agonized and some joyous, eventually one feels there is, metaphorically, a light at the end of the tunnel. One could take that,' he suggested, 'as a scenario of some phase of someone's life, which, as a variation among others, could have had as its original theme, the sequence of events at birth.'

Dr Laing wonders why obstetricians are reluctant to consider the child as a sensitive being, and the most specific question he throws into the arena is why, in normal delivery, it has now become the custom to cut the umbilical cord before it has finished pulsating naturally.

When the baby is first delivered, the cord is wet and pulsating. As soon as his air passages have been gently sucked out to make sure there is no mucous or other liquid to block his breathing the normal medical practice is to lay him on a flat surface, where the doctor can get at him easily, and a clamp is put on the cord about six inches from his navel. Another clamp is put on the cord about three inches closer to the mother. Then the cord is cut in between the clamps. Severed by steel. Which is fine, if it is not before the time it stops pulsating of its own accord.

Unfortunately the speedy efficiency of our hospitalized births are giving the cord, and the babies, a rough time. Although it was a common practice to leave the baby lying alongside the mother, with the cord intact until it finished pulsating, doctors now usually snip off that piece of living flesh, as though it were already dead. It is quite possible that this shock after the exertions of labour, may accentuate trauma for the child.

It takes about five minutes for the baby's own circulation to become established. Leaving the cord, instead of cutting it immediately, gives an overlap of time while the baby is still receiving oxygen via the cord. The lungs take over as the child inhales. The old blood vessel transporting oxygen to him (the umbilical life cord) gradually seals off as the new system takes over. This is the logical time to make the cut.

At the I.S.P.O.G. conference, Dr Laing related the story of his own birth and explained the effect he believes the hasty cutting of the cord had on his infant being.

'I can remember it happening to me as a body blow, a searing pain, a complete total organismic reflex, unguarded by any segmentalization, which took my breath away before I got my breath, and produced a triple red light, emotional, physical, and mental state of emergency and danger. Quite suddenly the only status quo I knew was, within seconds—the time it took for scissors and clamp to sever that connection—abruptly ended. It happened just after being born, which could be regarded as out of the frying pan into the fire. Being born was an experience I certainly wouldn't like to repeat.'

He pointed out that in some parts of the world the cord is left until the placenta comes out and then, with placenta and cord still attached, the naked baby is placed against the naked body of the mother.

'They all seem to be quite happy,' he said. 'And I would like to know why in our society the cord might not be left to be cut until as late as possible, rather than as quickly as possible? In psycho-analytic experience, a great deal of emphasis has been given to original traumatic situations. Freud took trauma to be a situation where input was beyond being handled or processed in the ordinary manner, because it was overwhelming. I would think that cutting the cord before breathing has been established is an extremely traumatic situation.

The emphasis which has been put on castration and mutilation anxieties is ante-dated by the traumatic experience of births where this cutting has been done; where a whole continuum has been severed before the physiological, biologic timing has been announced by the phasing out of the umbilical circulation and the natural closing of the heart valves. What I feel from my own physical memory is that there was an enormous confused shunning and panic going on around the cardiac region. I think it takes a long while to get over. If ever.'

Dr Laing is prepared to grant that these memories could be false, could be something in the nature of hallucinations; but by the same token so could memories of yesterday, so that it becomes a question of defining memory and judging variable individual experience. Simply to ponder the validity of certain obstetric practices opens up endless vistas.

'The obstetrician,' he says, 'has to think of the father, the other children, the mother, and the infant being born as a fully paid up member of the family, another limb of the octopus, as a sentient being, I would suggest an exquisitely sentient being, even more sensitive than we are.'

At the same conference Professor Norman Morris, M.D., F.R.C.O.G., consultant gynaecologist to the Obstetric Division of the Charing Cross Hospital, London, and President of the International Society of Psychosomatic Obstetrics and Gynaecology, said that his own daughter maintained she could remember being born and seeing 'a blinding white light' as she came out into the open. He said: 'It seems to me that babies from the moment of birth are very much more people than we as obstetricians and our colleagues as paediatricians have always appreciated. In other words, because they can't talk back to us we think their sensory systems are inadequate.' Another obstetrician made the point that most of the people in the room were 'practical people concerned with the business of living'. He said, 'I'm grateful to Dr Laing if he has repeated the awareness of the necessity to regard the individual baby not as a "something" but as a person.'

And a midwife who said she used to bend over the children of her deliveries until the cord finished pulsating, so that it would not be cut too soon and the baby could still feel a warm body near, said that although doctors sometimes objected, she managed to do this with twenty out of every twenty-three babies. The twenty would stop crying and be at ease, the other three were, in her words, 'inconsolable'.

I don't want my babies to be inconsolable. It sounds so final, so sad. It seems to me, unless there is a respiratory problem, that if there is any possibility of alleviating the trauma surrrounding birth by something as simple as leaving the cord intact until it has finished its work naturally, then it must be worth bringing it up with your own doctor. See what he has to say about it. Ask him to consider the baby. Say you do not want the cord to be cut until it is ready. This unique bond between you and your baby should be left to complete its cycle. It may take longer and it may be less convenient, especially in hospital delivery, but if it may also be physically and psychologically beneficial to the child, it is worth pleading the cause of non-violence in obstetrics. The natural timing of the umbilical link enables the blood to drain through, the pulsation to cease, the child's lungs to be fully prepared for the task of maintaining independent life, before the cord is cut. As Dr Laing says, we have to consider the first experiences of the senses in the world outside the uterus. As a doctor and a psychiatrist, he is qualified to assess as well as anyone whether or not this could be when first programming occurs. His view is that: 'Sequences in these first few seconds are going to provide us with the inner core, the basic tone, like the inner part of the onion. If we consider the senses of taste, touch, sound, sight and smell, the way a baby is treated in these first few moments is, in most places, an unmitigated disaster. It is difficult to think of a worse way to deal with a newborn baby and hard to imagine it done any worse than it's done now.

'The natural protective viscid covering of the skin, the vernix, which provides a buffer from the air and maintains a continuum, not only of nutrition but comfort and sensibility with the intrauterine environment, is wiped off, and raw red skin exposed, which is then dusted with dry talcum powder. The eyes are wiped and drops of silver nitrate put in, which is more than unpleasant, an intense caustic substance which no adult would like to put in his eyes, a prophylactic against venereal infection of the eye, which is put in routinely, whether the mother protests or not.

'Then the first thing which is put into the nose is a rubber tube which goes right down into the laryngeal passage, or dwells above it, and a suction pump is turned on which sucks mucus out of the lungs, because, supposedly, it has no business being there—although I don't know what on earth happened for the millions of years before suction pumps were invented . . . then the suction is reversed and air is pumped into the lungs, blown in like a bicycle tyre.

'After that cutting and wiping and dusting, a baby is picked up, wrapped up and bundled off to special segregated sterilized environments, away from the mother. Separated from her vibrations, from her bio-electric field, from her smell, from all physical contact with her, and handled for the first hours through rubber or plastic, a teat and bottle may be proffered by any nurse who happens to be on duty; the baby is then wrapped in materials which are the replacement for the womb environment.'

Much of Dr Laing's work and therapy now is centred around the birth experience and its effects. One of the customs to which he drew attention in a seminar on birth,[1] was that practised in northern India, whereby such minute care is taken with the baby's first experience of taste, for instance, that the family astrologer works out the gem or metal relevant to the constellations and planetary influences in evidence at the moment of birth, and then a finely ground powder of that metal is mixed with honey, and placed on the tip of the lip and the tongue of the baby, so ensuring the benign nature of a child's first taste of extra-uterine life. There is no comparable consideration given to the senses of the newborn in most of western civilization. In Dr Laing's opinion this extraordinary insensitivity towards the newborn is reflected in mankind's present desire to run from nature, the prevailing feeling that by being an element that cannot always be controlled, nature is frightening.

Our own first experiences at birth may set patterns to which we are eternally bound. Without seeing it, we dance to that first tune, look for the same taste, repeat the sequence of our first worldly relationship, that of mother and child. Our experience of other people goes back to our experience of our mother. If there is separation, then there will either be the wish for reunion, or the wish to maintain separation, distance, lack of expression and feeling. As Dr Laing says, the residue of the dynamics of that early drama is in our present life, and if it was catastrophic, might we not then unconsciously precipitate the tragedy over and over again in our adult relationships? These evocations from the past manifest themselves again and again as adult disturbance.

If we wait to cut the cord, we may improve the quality of birth and life.

Don't Slap Your Baby into Life: Dr Frederick Leboyer

The simple suggestion to leave the umbilical cord until it finishes pulsating is put into practical effect by a French doctor, Frederick

1. London, 17th October, 1972.

Leboyer, who, in the past few years of his practice as an obstetrician, has come to the conclusion that too little sensitivity is shown towards newly born babies. He has developed a step-by-step method of soothing the infant's first moments outside the womb. He says it is an *attitude* towards birth rather than a technique—put the baby first!

For nine months you have prepared yourself for this moment. Now your baby is born. If he breathes spontaneously, leave him alone. Don't slap him into life. Don't hang him by his heels and shake him. He doesn't have to cry to show he's alive. Love him into life, as you loved him into existence. Your baby is a human being. His sensitivity now is unequalled at any other time. Putting his well-being first will affect the rest of his life.

French doctors have long been famous for their care of the woman in pregnancy and labour. Now it's the baby's turn. Dr Leboyer is a small, soft-spoken man of radical views whose work in considering the baby at birth has made obstetricians and midwives all over the world sit up and take notice.[1] In France, medical colleagues were affronted by his implied attack on established methods of delivering babies. Even women themselves have taken time to accept the idea that the focus of attention should move from mother to infant once labour is complete.

Now retired, and living in India for two months of each year, Frederick Leboyer has spent most of his life as a busy obstetrician with a private clinic in Paris, which is where he developed his technique for delivering babies in the most harmonious circumstances possible.

I talked to him when he came to London to show the film of one of his deliveries, and he made it clear that he wants us to think of the baby as we would of an adult, to credit the newborn with sensibility and sensitivity, to accept and pay attention to the fact that being born is a 'raw state' in which to be, and that our adult awareness of this must lead us to help and cosset the child.

He says that technically a newborn infant is hypersensitive through the skin, the eyes and the ears. Coming out of the constriction of the womb and then the birth canal, the child should be able to feel joy and relief at this new freedom and space, rather than immediately being restricted again by businesslike bundling into

1. *Birth Without Violence*, published in France, 1974; U.S.A. and England, 1975. He has also made a documentary film, *A Child is Born*.

clothes, and onto scales. After some nine thousand deliveries, Leboyer began to wonder why babies always seemed to sob when they were born.

'I am interested in the significance and origin of suffering,' he told me, 'not in the medical sense of "fetal suffering", but emotional pain. The despair and the sorrow.'

He decided that some of it is attributable to the infant's violent experiences while being born, but is convinced that one of the prime causes is the lack of understanding with which the newborn is welcomed into the world, and he now wants birth to be made more bearable. A natural progression of events takes place in his delivery room, which provides simple precautions against giving the baby unnecessary jolts in the first moments of earthlife.

To begin with he delivers babies in subdued light to shield their eyes, and near silence to protect their ears.

In watching the film of a delivery in his Paris clinic, the greatest impact is the sound of silence. The first murmurings of the baby's voice come through like music. There is no shocked squall of awakening, no clatter and bustle of the usual harshly lit delivery room, no busy officials separating the ritual into efficient compartments.

Leboyer's delivery techniques were worked out as he looked for a way to make the transition from internal to external life more gradual and less shocking, by prolonging some of the sensations a baby feels in the uterus, and by introducing the baby to new ones slowly.

All our life, energy runs through the spine, but during birth people forget that a baby's spine is too delicate and tender to be jerked upside down as so often happens when a baby is taken by the heels and smacked into taking its first breath. So Leboyer avoids handling the baby roughly. He allows the child to be born, if it is a normal labour, in the soothing half-dark. He makes a point of leaving the umbilical cord to finish pulsating, as advocated by Dr Laing. Dr Leboyer maintains that air burns as it goes down the nose and throat of a newborn infant, and leaving the cord gives the baby time to adjust to air by letting him continue to receive oxygen through the blood pulsating in the cord as he has done for his time in the womb.

Leboyer takes into consideration both the physical and emotional effects of cutting the cord too soon. He says that physically it could cause oxygen deprivation and emotionally the separation from the mother's body is too sudden and too shocking. So, while waiting to cut the cord, he first gives the baby to the mother to hold to her stomach and breast. Neither child nor mother is dressed, so their first contact is skin to skin, heart to heart. The doctor's reasoning is that clothes would feel scorching to new skin and the only bearable texture for such tenderness is the softness of the maternal skin touch.

He instructs the mother to put her hands on the baby's back to hold him to her; or the contact could be through the father's hands or the doctor's. There should be a kind of gentle massage, so that the child can feel warmth and security with his first experience of human manipulation.

Lastly the baby is put slowly into a warm bath, so returning to his accustomed environment, liquid. He is not scrubbed with soap, but held lightly so that he regains the sensation of weightlessness that he knew in the womb. His eyes are open, he is breathing quietly, his limbs stretch out. Instead of screams and the pain of severance, there is calm. He has survived the hazards of gestation and the turbulence of birth. The baby begins life being touched by his parents and playing in water.

I know that when my babies were born, the first thing I wanted to do was touch them and hold them; I wanted to push away instruments and strangers; I wanted time to adjust to having borne a new life, and time for the child to adjust to being with me but outside me, to being in air, to touching the hands of his father and knowing our presence.

All the evidence of experience and common sense point to the importance of the way a child's moments of birth are handled. Leboyer is eager to avoid labels, saying that we are drowning in 'techniques', and reiterates over and over again that the vital point is our 'attitude' to birth.

Attitudes towards newborn children have to begin with the women who are bearing them and the men who have fathered them. Hopefully they will be backed up by the men and women, the doctors and nurses who have chosen the job of birth attendants. Doctors who believe in change, like Leboyer and Laing, may slowly bring the medical establishment to intellectual awareness of the truths of nature. Parents are the people who could and should begin to do something about manifesting them in their own lives and the lives of their children. So we must understand the message correctly.

Advocating harmony at birth does not mean the sacrifice of safety. Neither child nor mother, as Leboyer is careful to point out, must ever be allowed to go short of oxygen. A complicated or abnormal delivery cannot take place in half-light. Fetal or maternal distress must be watched for and taken care of. But the essence of this procedure is that it is based on an attitude towards birth, and deals with alleviating fear in the newborn, so that the first thing we experience in life is not something so terrible that it blocks out early memory, as it has for most of us.

Vital to Leboyer's birth attitude must be a woman's own attitude to her body, her baby and her birth-giving. Only with her participation, her calm, her lack of fear, her aware state of consciousness, will the method really work. She will not be able to massage her own child if she is slumped half-unconscious from drugs, she will not be able to help deliver the baby if she does not know how to work with contractions, and a forceps delivery to an unrelaxed or drugged mother hardly constitutes a gentle welcome for the child, however well-meaning the obstetrician may be.

So let's try to make being born a little easier on our babies. Let's really prepare ourselves for their coming, and try to communicate with them straight away. By easing the violence of birth we may help defuse the violence of life.

At the end of Leboyer's film the baby he has delivered is radiating calm and peace with open eyes and a beamy smile. The only time he made a sound was as the cord was cut and he was taken away from his mother. A child does not have to cry before he can breathe. He can see and feel and hear and smile. If he's happy.

Think How It Feels To Be Born: Prof. Elizabeth Fehr

Profound theories on the effect of the birth trauma have been developed at length and depth by the great psychologists and psychiatrists of our time. Carl Jung, Sigmund Freud, Otto Rank, Theodor Reik, Wilhelm Reich, and now R. D. Laing, have had their own specific theses on how and why birth affects us so deeply and sets up patterns of behaviour for our entire lives, unless something is done to change the imprint.

Something can be done. It is the experience of some psychologists that initial birth impressions can be erased by taking patients back to their own birth experiences to relive being born. The problem is how do we prevent a traumatic birth traumatizing us for the rest of our lives? The answers are that for the generations born in pain, their haunting memory of it can be alleviated by bringing it from the unconscious to the conscious mind. But for the generations to come it may be possible to side-step the pain altogether. We can think and feel for the child as he is born. We can care about the way he is first handled, the feelings he first comes in contact with.

Think of that tiny vulnerable creature making his way out of your narrow passage, suddenly pushed by a force beyond himself, into a place beyond his comprehension; out of the floaty warmth of you, into air. Try to play 'being born' yourself. You will see how it could be for a baby. Simulating the experience may fill out the shadows and give some present reality to a forgotten feeling.

Submerge your head in the bath, eyes and mouth closed, ears completely under water. Even the smallest noise from your intestine resounds in a giant roar. If you open your mouth to yawn it is like an avalanche; if you fart it is a volcano erupting; speaking, let alone wailing, is more like a thunderstorm than a voice.

This seems to me the way a baby might hear his mother's sounds while he is still in the womb. I am sure most doctors will argue that any sound would be thoroughly muffled, if indeed the baby could hear at all, because an unborn baby's eardrum is completely surrounded by liquid, whereas in an adult the eardrum is surrounded by air. The conflicting view is that babies not only hear in the womb and the birth canal, but hear clearly. My own feeling is that if in fact it has been found that unborn babies hear something, then whatever it is will be their first experience of sound, and those sounds are likely to register on the sensitive unborn system with all the magnitude of the unknown.

So try to imagine, wetly, how it might be in the womb as labour is beginning. You are surrounded by liquid. Each gurgle reverberates. You begin to work your way out, trying to push through a narrow constricting passage. Suddenly the normal noises of your mother's internal life system become more exaggerated. The walls of the canal you've been trying to navigate heave against you, the motion getting stronger and stronger. Your mother's labour lament howls through you like an electric shock clanging and banging in your head. The volume and intensity is terrifying.

Take that little ball of feeling, that microcosm reflecting the macrocosm of humanity. If you are alone and afraid, how does he sense your fear and your isolation? How deeply might that tamper with his innermost balance, perhaps tip the scale between stability and instability, confidence and inhibition? How *does* he experience the alienation of sterile hospital wards; the metallic clang of instruments; the intrusion of the strange, separation from the known? Maybe the only way to blot out that terror, that shock, is to attempt total forgetfulness. Maybe it is not possible to forget, only to suppress.

You may think we will never know the answers to these questions. But once questions are asked, and continue to be asked, eventually a glimmer of understanding begins to emerge. In the same way that doctors and scientists are now researching the effects of all the machines they have created, the drugs they have concocted, the routines they have invented—so too psychologists and psychiatrists are beginning to find out what happens to our minds in the earliest, most receptive part of our lives. On the whole it is now recognized that babies not only feel while they are being born, but they hear.[1] The child not only registers sound while he is in your belly, but the sounds are enormously magnified so that what he hears as he is pushing down the birth passage is imprinted onto his brain and carried into future life.[2]

There is also clear evidence that immediately after birth, the newborn baby can not only turn to sound, but also localize smell and therefore have an auditory and visual co-ordination. He also shows the expectation that sound comes from the mouth and he can adjust to distance.[3]

Virginia Johnson, a woman psychologist working with schizophrenics in Los Angeles, has discovered that by taking people back to their earliest experiences of life under the influence of a drug called methylphenidate[4] they could actually recall the first few weeks of life. In 1971, she reported at the second meeting of the Society for Neuroscience in Houston, Texas, that this kind of recall gave clear indication that 'neonatal experiences were frequently related to

1. *Science News*, p. 313, U.S.A., 11th June, 1971.
2. *Science News*, p. 263, U.S.A., 21st October, 1972.
3. *Journal of Genetic Psychology*, Vol. 66, p. 281. And *Archives of Disease in Childhood*, 1961, Vol. 36, p. 50.
4. *Science News*, p. 313, U.S.A., 11th June, 1971.

psychopathological symptoms seen later in life', and suggested that some of these early experiences might lead to schizophrenia. She based her concept on analysis of taped interviews with people representing a wide range of psychopathological syndromes.[1]

She found that common symptoms of schizophrenia, most particularly those known as 'auditory hallucinations'—hearing voices when there is apparently no one there—directly correlate with an altered state of consciousness shortly before or shortly after birth. The altered state of consciousness is caused by shock, acute pain, fever, concussion and anoxia (lack of oxygen). She thinks schizophrenia reflects an auditory memory of something first experienced in the womb or the birth canal, and because babies can hear during pregnancy and hear even more clearly during the traumatic trip through the birth canal, the secret voices of 'madness' may be the repetition of sounds heard while being born.

Her point is that there are certain high-risk factors that could be avoided; for instance, conditions which might contribute towards dysfunction in the central nervous system of the fetus during the last few weeks of pregnancy, traumatic labour and delivery, and complications in the period immediately after birth, such as emergency surgery, drug reactions and toxicity.

Professor Elizabeth Fehr, who died suddenly in the spring of 1974 at the age of fifty-three, was an American psychologist who had been working in New York on the theory that traumatic birth can hold children back for the rest of their lives and actually affect physical as well as emotional development.

In the preceding five years she had worked on a technique which she called 'rebirthing', taking you back to your own birth experience. It simulates being back in the womb, moving through the birth canal and out into the world again.

Professor Fehr believed that once an area of obstruction had been pinpointed, the obstruction could then be released. By using what she called 'Natal Therapy' to help people recall their birth experiences, she herself could see the area in which they became 'stuck' or obstructed during labour and delivery. According to her experiments, the obstruction can be relieved through a process of reconstructing as nearly as possible the physical sensations of being born. If the rebirthing is done under affectionate relaxed circumstances, the adult

1. *Science News*, p. 263, 21st October, 1972.

is also freed from having continually to act out his birth traumas, because this time there is no anaesthetic, no instruments, no interference, but a loving welcome.

It was discovered by Professor Fehr that rebirthing helped her subjects cross physical barriers that she believed to be an intrinsic part of the cause of mental disorder. Her thesis on the effects and cure of birth trauma was being developed under her supervision by a group known as A.I.M.E., the Analytical Institute for Motivational Education, in New York City. Each member of the community has been through natal therapy, reliving their birth several times, and each claims total recall of the original experience.

Professor Fehr was herself a mother and grandmother. For sixteen years she was married to a physician and during that time studied medicine, helping with her husband's lectures and research. She also went through a nurse's training and worked as a nurse in her husband's private practice. Her death came while she was in the middle of experimental work with her daughter Leslie. They were together exploring the possibility that natal therapy taps the non-verbal hemisphere of the brain and facilitates transfer of unconscious material to the conscious mind, thus achieving, without drugs, much the same effect as Virginia Johnson—absolute recall of the birth experience. Leslie is continuing her mother's development of natal therapy at the Institute of Natal Therapy, New York.[1]

Elizabeth Fehr held an Associate Professorship in Human Relations and was a New York State certified psychotherapist. She had been working in therapy for fourteen years when I first met her, but considered herself more a teacher than an analyst. She was trained at the Post Graduate Center for Mental Health in New York and after eleven years became a member of the teaching staff. She first worked in social therapy, dealing with those who had just come out of mental hospitals, then in poetry therapy, then psychotherapy. She went through her own analysis with a psychiatrist, standard procedure in becoming a qualified therapist; took her own group therapy sessions and then 'professional' group therapy sessions which were specifically for members of the medical profession.

After receiving an Honorary Professorship, Mrs Fehr went into private practice in New York. The idea of 'rebirthing' came through

1. The Institute of Natal Therapy, 3 East 80th Street, New York 10021.

an experience with one of her patients, a young man in his early twenties, who was painfully sensitive about his height, which was only five feet five inches. One day, while in session with her, he told her he felt as though he was trying to get out of a manhole, but couldn't wriggle through. He started pushing himself up from the arms of his chair. She recognized it as a re-enactment of the birth trauma, and started to help him through the invisible hole by pushing him herself, adding her strength to his, and in so doing, she herself became the mother, pushing him out through her own psychic and physical energy.

'We went on pushing together,' she told me, 'until he was out. Boy, was he stuck!'

So stuck that they went round the room, along the corridors and into the street before he was out. Since then he has grown more than two inches taller. That was only the beginning for Professor Fehr's work in this direction. A girl who had worn thick-lensed spectacles all her life in an attempt to cope with being unable to see in three dimensions, could throw off her glasses after being rebirthed. For several days she didn't need them at all. Now she has much weaker lenses, sees three-dimensionally, and believes she will be able to throw them away completely one day.

Elizabeth Fehr's experimental work began in 1969, and by mid-1970 she had 'birthed' about six people. Due to the consistent and dramatic results of her work, she formulated the therapy officially and went on to 'birth' an increasing number of patients. 'I took all those patients I was working with in my practice and went with them right back through their birth experiences. By sharing the intensity of this they became very close. Like a family.'

This group of people became the A.I.M.E. Community, with Mrs Fehr its matriarchal head. They worked and lived together in communal houses in her lifetime, although since her death the Community has dissolved. One woman who had limped all her life, a defect for which doctors could find no reason and no cure, found the cause of it through working with Professor Fehr. During her rebirth she could feel something holding back her damaged foot. She says she felt another presence there, as though someone were clasping her foot and wouldn't let go.

This led her back to her own mother and questions about being born. It turned out that she had been an identical twin, although no one had told her so because her sister was stillborn. Her own foot had become entangled with a limb of the dead fetus. The permanent affliction she had lived with was the buried memory of her dead sister, born after her, trying to hold on.

Professor Fehr's diagnosis was that rebirthing, however difficult, 'brought it out into the open and finally relieved her of the unconscious burden of something she had not been allowed to formulate or admit consciously.'

'It is rehabilitation,' said Elizabeth Fehr. 'Forming a bridge back to life.'

I was introduced to Professor Fehr by an English psychiatrist in London in the hot summer of 1973. She was in London to demonstrate her technique to a group of aggressively sceptical psychiatrists, their students and patients.

Disbelieving, but curious, I watched her work and was unable to resist the experiment. I remembered nothing about my birth and seriously doubted the possibility of such a memory ever being rekindled. But it did seem right to me that a child could feel during its birth, and that those feelings might alter its pattern through life.

So I was my own guinea pig. Even against my conscious will, I was drawn into the experiment.

I lay on a foam-rubber mattress twenty foot long in a large flat in Maida Vale. The mattress represented the birth canal, and was foam for comfort since the subjects had to travel along it as they had their mother's vagina. On either side live bodies pressed against me, simulating the contracting walls of the uterus.

The technique for recalling my own birth went like this:

Professor Fehr bent over me, clasping my hands, telling me to breathe in and out to my own most comfortable rhythm, as one does at the beginning of labour in fact. I used level A (see Appendix I) and maintained eye contact with her.

'Close your eyes,' she said.

Lids closed, I begin imagining how it might feel to be inside a womb. A visual image flashes in, as though I am squashed into a red kaleidoscope. Is this a consciously constructed image or an unconscious memory? Too conscious. I'm still thinking. Still breathing in and out, in and out. Hands begin to push me. In return my muscles tense. The movement seems to push me along the passage. I don't hear voices in the room any more. I don't know what's happening. I'm not in control of what's happening any more. I can feel my mother. I can feel her presence all round me. Can sense her as a girl. Feel her frightened. Feel her lonely. Threatened. Feel myself quite strong. Wanting to reassure her. Not knowing if I called out. Feeling excruciating pain in my stomach and my back. Like a steel girdle. Distantly hear someone saying, 'She's stuck there, she's stuck—try to get out, Danaë, try and get out of it.'

I was stuck. Struggling to relieve that pain. Fighting and kicking like a horse to get out of that immovable vice round my hips. Kicking my feet out. And bouncing up as I did it. Straight up. Sitting. The strain gone. Infinite relief.

Afterwards, after my rebirthing, I felt the closeness of my mother and the absence of my father like a loss, lingering with me a long time. Knowing my father was not there, and recognizing a sadness I had felt before, but not knowing its origin.

Later, I asked my mother about how I was born and she explained that it was during the war. My father had been away fighting. She was alone in her house with only a nurse, no doctor. The nurse wouldn't let her light a fire in her room, and she was waiting for her mother to come, but she didn't. She said it was awful and lonely and she was very frightened. She hadn't wanted to tell me about it before, because it seemed pointless. I felt that closeness from the rebirthing reinforced.

When I got home that night, it wasn't time for my period and I am very regular, but I was pouring with blood.

Now I not only feel my mother in a slightly different, more understanding way, as a woman. But I realize where my original fear of giving birth may have come from. And the agonizing backaches I have been getting all my life have almost completely disappeared. Whatever Elizabeth Fehr's experiments might have meant to others, to me she gave back part of the memory of being born.

Her work has brought into focus the serious setbacks that can be caused by obstetrical interference during labour and delivery. She found that children born with excessive intervention in the natural rhythm of labour have strong psychological as well as physical handicaps. According to her theories, instrument babies tend to be dissatisfied because they 'didn't get born by themselves'.

She explained: 'They weren't permitted to finish by themselves a process they had begun, so for the rest of their lives they are either having to prove to themselves and the world that they can do everything by themselves. Or they can do nothing without help. If babies have interference to the head, or get "stuck" in the head, I call them "head babies". They are strictly "head" people. The emotional system needs reawakening. It can't keep up with the intellect.'

It turned out that John, my husband, was just such a case. When he was rebirthed by Elizabeth, I heard him yell at those pushing him along the birth canal, 'Get off my head! Get off my head!' But there was no one near his head. Afterwards he said, 'I felt as though someone's hand was pressing down on my skull so I couldn't move.'

'That's where you were stuck,' said Elizabeth.

In fact John did have a forceps delivery—his mother's pelvis is minute, and as a baby his head was particularly big. He suffered from severe migraine in childhood. He is wary of showing his deeper emotions. So much so that until his rebirthing, he hadn't shed a tear between early childhood and the day his son was born. Since the rebirthing his mysterious headaches have gone—and he cried at a television documentary!

Labours induced for no specific medical reason can cause a child to have lasting feelings of having been pushed out before being ready. Not in his own time. 'They have a fury that endures through life,' said Professor Fehr. 'They feel as though they have been dispossessed—livid they were not given the time to come out as and when they wanted.'

The result is children who feel unwanted—thrown out—not loved or understood. They have to have everything their own way to compensate in later life. 'To the point of real nuttiness,' said Elizabeth in her usual blunt way. 'If they don't get their own way, the stubbornness turns to rage.'

Babies who wanted to come out buttocks first, the breech position, and were manually turned, also harbour huge resentments, she said.

'Again,' she explained 'they weren't permitted to do what they wanted to do, so they're furious. They didn't get their way, so for the rest of their lives they have to at any cost, or they're completely defeated, knowing they cannot.'

Professor Fehr reiterated the importance of relaxation in the woman. 'A reassured mother can make all the difference. Many people who experience their births again, scream. That's not their scream, it's the mother's scream they are acting out. They are still attached to her so they hear it, feel it, know it.

'To many children whose mothers were heavily sedated, the rest of their lives seem unreal. They didn't have any experience of being born, so from then on everything is fake. Some women simply will not contemplate pain. They say "put me out" without thinking that the baby is "out" too. So both have missed the experience of a lifetime. There is a sense of loss for ever more.'

The success of Elizabeth Fehr's work supports my belief that children feel how they are being born while they are being born. And now I am convinced it makes a difference to the child. If the mother feels frightened, lonely and threatened, there's every chance the child will too. If the mother is tense, the child may have to fight to get out, fight for its life.

We can't turn our backs on those vulnerable wombchildren and pretend that our behaviour doesn't affect them. It appears that human beings have developed a reflex to remove pain memories. Since birth has been obliterated in almost all our minds it leads one to imagine that it might have been pretty horrific. And it leads me to think there are things which could and should be done about it. Changing our whole attitude to birth, replacing expediency with tenderness, machines and devices with loving people, could substantially change the impact of their first moments on the future lives of our children.

* * *

When I was having my children, and immediately after their birth, I was sharply aware of how extraordinary, yet ordinary, is the process of giving birth. Everyone is in some way touched by it, whether they have children of their own or not. Somewhere in the mind of each one of us is a recollection of being born, whether it comes to the surface and becomes focused or not. Almost all of us know at some time some one who is giving birth. The degree of involvement with this biological, spiritual and emotional event varies with the individual.

I first began writing about birth because I felt so deeply that it was an experience to be shared; that when it was positive, it was miraculous, and miracles, or the possibility of them, should be accessible to as many people as they can be. I wrote from my emotions and was surprised at how much poured onto the paper.

Then I began seriously to consider the ripples which spread out from my own experience of giving birth, and preparing for birth. If I was to stick my neck out and urge that women give themselves the opportunity to be alive to the birth of their children, that men allow them to take that opportunity and try to share in it too, that world consciousness of birth be altered to encompass the feelings of parents and babies, then I was going to have to go into the socio-logical, medical, biological and practical reality of my emotional statement.

Once started on that venture, it was almost impossible to stop. Every time I turned a stone, I uncovered some new and amazing fact. Sometimes it was a pleasant surprise, sometimes very alarming. The first part of this book has set down my ideal, which is to make sure in a scientific age that nature is allowed to function as it should for the birth of a child, and that technology is used to help only in cases of emergency. Hopefully this thought has aroused some awarenesses about being born and giving birth that have been buried by the mechanized life-styles of today; hopefully you can relate to things I have said enough to want to know how we can make a reality of this ideal, taking into account both the factors which have always existed, like the way our bodies work and new lives are created and brought forth; and those which are new and variable, like the inventions and techniques that spring up, like strange monsters, without giving us a chance to assess them before the next one comes ticking and clacking over the horizon.

You know now I believe that preparing women for birth in the most comprehensive way possible is the only chance we have to improve the conditions of birth for future generations. But the desire for this improvement has to come from all of us eventually—mothers, fathers, grandparents, doctors, nurses. Once the desire is established, there must be education, guidance, facts; practical tools to bring about change. Here then in Part II is a flexible practical structure for preparing yourselves to stay close to nature while giving birth in the machine age.

II

Naturebirth
A Practical Guide

NATUREBIRTH is conscious birth. To be conscious for birth, we need to be conscious in pregnancy; we need to know as much as possible about our bodies, our minds, and how they function together, both during the time a baby is forming in the womb and in the powerful movement and sensations of labour.

Essential to preparation for Naturebirth is a sense of the importance of immediate contact with nature as a way to understanding and integrating the spiritual and the physical self. Preparation offers information as an aid to achieving this total awareness.

This is not an admonition to return to the primitive as the only true way—but rather an admonition not to deny the primitive instincts which are in all of us; to blend ancient wisdom with new science, but to recognize that in calling either one absolute, there is always a margin of error. There is an element in nature for which we have no scientific explanation: the life force. It can neither be replaced by machinery nor controlled by it. Technology should abet the course of nature, yet there is evidence that man's mechanical interference is in danger of disturbing a fragile natural balance. In the last analysis, instinct may be as precise a guide as we ever have. Learning how to listen to, interpret and act upon instinct is a vital part of the preparation for Naturebirth. In acknowledging the validity of the instinctive impulse we allow ourselves the chance to feel birth at every level of consciousness.

5

Preparing Yourselves

How to Get Together Your Own Preparation Group

Here are some suggestions for how to set up your own groups for Naturebirth preparation. The guidance applies as much for two people as for ten, although the practical tips are geared to groups rather than couples only, since several people are a little more complicated to organize than two. The preparation is for mind and body, considered as inseparable and inextricable. There is food for thought and there are physical exercises to practise. The exercises are explained in detail in Appendix I, and the only hard and fast rule I would emphasize is the necessity for doing them as often as possible. Think of it as an athlete would, getting into training for a big event. He has to work to be ready for it. You have to work to be ready for birth.

So first let us say that the gathering of people in like condition should be informal. This is not a school class. You are getting together to learn about birth. You want to prepare yourselves in the best way you can so that having a baby can mean good times, instead of being a miserable exile to some place of weighty gloom. It is going to involve hard work, on yourself, and on each other, so the room in which you choose to meet becomes both a work room and a play room.

Ideally it should be light and bright with plenty of space. There should be large windows to let in fresh air and sunlight. The best place to sit for exercises is on the floor, so try to collect enough big, supportive cushions for people to sit on and lean against comfortably. The specific skill to be learned, conscious controlled breathing under stress, requires that you be upright, relaxed and comfortable, so it's usually easiest to sit on the floor, leaning against a wall, but cushioned by pillows. This is the best position for labour too, so sitting in this way prepares you for dealing with real contractions.

There will be new awarenesses to be unearthed. Preparation draws attention to the way babies are formed; how they grow inside a woman and how that affects glands which in turn secrete hormones to alter the intricate balance of emotional responses; how valuable the support of other women can be at such a time, and how important it is for men and women to share the whole process of pregnancy, labour and delivery, if they have deliberately chosen to have children together.

You need to know about yourselves, your feelings, your approach to birth, and to be fully prepared you need facts about the mechanical devices, drugs and attitudes you are likely to encounter. There must be space in which to learn all this, willingness to face mistakes, start all over again, change your approach if necessary, learn from each other. Space to practise all the exercises, over and over again, so that you are not just playing a game with yourself as you wait for a miracle to drop into your lap, but are working towards a specific end.

The details of how each particular group functions will inevitably vary from one to another. There are certain things to decide on, such as how long a session will last, what time it will begin, where it will take place, how many people should be included and how much each should contribute for teaching aids, drinks or extra pillows.

The easiest thing is for everyone to work out these details among themselves, according to their individual needs and means. Money has to be found to buy teaching aids, if you want them, and someone will have to offer a room once a week—or perhaps once a fortnight to begin with. We have found it important that there be a fair exchange in terms of energy and money—otherwise there is usually someone who feels put upon. There is always a balanced rate of exchange, and it is important to find it and agree to the terms of your meetings before you start preparation. The last thing you want is sniping and bitchiness to creep into the atmosphere. It is just a question of establishing a flexible structure and not letting things slide until someone gets uptight. We find that to ask for and to pay about £1.50 or $3.00 seems reasonable to everyone concerned. But that obviously has to go up, or down, in relation to the general cost of living, and how much money you can spare.

I suggest that if you are in a group, approximately two hours should be set aside for a preparation session. Where groups are to include men and women who work during the day, find a time in the evening after everyone has had a chance to relax a little. As a general rule, there should be one class early in pregnancy, say the fourth month, to prime you for what is to come, and then a systematic covering of all necessary information (and that does change quite rapidly when you are considering obstetric techniques and equipment, so try to keep up to date with the newest information available), and practice of the exercises, starting nearer the birth time, say the sixth or seventh month of pregnancy, once a week for eight or ten weeks. If you find you've gone through the whole thing long before the baby is born, then it is a good idea to have a little refresher session as near as possible to the date the baby is due. If each woman begins approximately eight weeks before the baby is due, she should attend one session every week. Groups rarely go above eight people because the gathering becomes too diffuse and concentration and communication more difficult. It's a good idea to start sessions in the morning because then everyone will come to it fresh and relaxed.

On the other hand, when my husband and I go through preparation with couples, we sometimes find it more convenient to meet in the evenings. Part of the reason for this is that we like to work with men and women, since my husband is so enthusiastic about the subject, and men are less hesitant to share the experience and their feelings about it with other men than in a purely female gathering. Since most of us work, evenings are the only time we can all get together. We aim to eat a light early supper, give ourselves time to ease off the hassles of the day, and have tea, coffee, juices or wine during the evening.

I think the best time for women to start preparation is in the seventh month of pregnancy. At that stage, you begin to see and feel the baby inside you, and there is plenty of time to practise the exercises. When I was pregnant with Orion, I started much later than this, in fact I was already eight months pregnant, so I did a kind of crash course in those last few weeks, practising the exercises hard every day and having sessions with Sara at least twice a week. If you are late turning onto the whole idea of preparation, it is possible to learn all there is to learn quickly. If you are ready to begin once you

119

know you are pregnant, there is nothing to stop you preparing from that moment on. One of the advantages of starting early is that men who want to take an active part in the process of preparation and birth can share even the earliest moments of pregnancy.

Set the scene to be as friendly and welcoming as possible. I remember one of the great things about Sara's sessions, both when I was seeing her alone before Orion's birth, and during the longer preparation for Liam when there were several other men and women present, was the peaceful environment. You could feel a sigh of relief as each person walked into the calm white room strewn with cushions. It was as if the burdens of daily life and the world outside the womb and that room simply lifted off and disappeared, so each of us became lighter, brighter, more relaxed and at the same time more alert.

We would sit on cushions on the floor, backs propped against a wall. We would put foam-rubber wedges covered in calico under our knees to help support the strain and extra weight of carrying our unborn babies. There were paintings on which to focus our eyes during breathing exercises. A shape or pattern of some kind on the wall is important. If you can follow something with your eyes, they don't become fixed and staring. Total relaxation includes the muscles of face and eyes.

Try to find a room with space, air, soft colours, plants. If you don't have a room like this or can't find one among friends and acquaintances, then just shove some furniture aside, take pillows off the beds, and don't be afraid to improvise. You can do it all outside, if the weather is good and you have the space. Do whatever you can to make the meeting place easy to be in, but make sure you do it before people arrive.

Make a point of having the windows open when practising breathing and muscle tone. Our bodies need more fuel to cope with our expanding bellies and the way muscles get fuel is through oxygen. Also of course, the baby needs it too. So, important as specific exercises are, it is good to get out into the open and walk as much as you can too.

Choosing a conductor, when you are in a group, or even if there are just two of you, ensures that exercises really get done. The conductor is in a special position of responsibility, so I have included some notes on the subject; and the exercises (explained in detail in Appendix I) are for muscle tone, dissociation, relaxation and breathing. You don't need to do them all at every session. Just see how the time goes and use common sense.

Thoughts for the Conductor:

The most important thing in the beginning is to have yourself together enough to go through the breathing exercises, checking each woman individually and encouraging each to do the pelvic floor and vaginal exercises as often as possible. The rest is simply bringing into focus as many topics as possible and guiding conversation so that the atmosphere is relaxed enough for discussions to be therapeutic. The most valuable and believable truth for anyone to learn from is your own personal experience.

Understanding oneself and one's own reaction to different situations works as a guide to others. Everyone is trying to learn how to cope most easily with the most difficult confrontations. If you already have some experience of birth, give it freely to your friends. It can do nothing but help them.

Then see that everyone is sitting comfortably, their backs well supported by cushions or pillows, their buttocks firmly on the ground. Start the relaxation exercise from the toes, and work up through the calves, knees, thighs, abdomen, chest, jaw, mouth, eyes. Ask them to tense up all the muscles involved, and then let go. Start again with the shoulders and work down the arms to the fingertips. Make sure they're completely aware of everything in their bodies and how it feels to clench and let go internal and external muscles. This lays the foundation for specific relaxation and breathing exercises and teaches awareness of the internal life of our bodies.

Remember not to let any of the exercises go on for too long and become tiring. About ten to fifteen minutes is the right amount of time to allow for practice of toning exercises. You will need longer, say at least half an hour a session, for the breathing. Exactly how long will probably vary with how well people are memorizing the different levels.

A preparation is a kind of ritual, and everything about it should be handled with care and sensitivity. You are getting ready for the rite of birth, a momentous event in human life. Pregnancy is the time you can take to clear your mind and the space around you. To use energy at source, in its highest, most positive form, the environment needs to be set in a way most conducive to receiving information. We utilize energy best in peace and calm.

I see birth itself as a magical act that brings forth life. It is logical to accord a certain respect to this time of preparation, as you would before any ceremony. For thousands of years pregnant women have been treated with special care. In the ancient civilizations of Egypt, China, Tibet and Greece, right through to the Renaissance in Europe it was considered crucial that a woman with child should become one with nature.

In the Middle Ages, the Rosicrucians, who were alchemists, the magicians of their time, believed absolutely that the environment into which a child was born, the one in which the mother lived during gestation, was vital to that child's development and affected its state of being for the rest of its life. They used nine-pointed stars to attract the moon's influence and surrounded their women with special herbs, scents, metals and 'sympathetic' figures. Even if there is no way to prove whether or not this affected the wombchild, it must have been soothing for the woman and that peace of mind must surely reflect on the child within.

The Greeks, too, practised what was known as 'eugenics', the science of 'producing fine offspring', where all possible precautions to maintain harmony were taken with women during pregnancy. The Mohammedans are more extreme: they believe in shutting women away completely before they give birth. But the point is the same— they wish the mother to be perfectly quiet, secure and free from interference. It is a time of sense and sensibility. A woman's senses become as fragile and acute as they may ever be, aware of the new and sensual life gradually developing its minute parts inside her.

I don't mean we should all immediately rush out to find magic talismans and scatter them round the house. You don't have to use nine-pointed stars to attract positive influence. Nor do we have to cut ourselves off from normal life. We can reinterpret those practices to suit the kind of lives we lead, bearing in mind that the underlying premise is to develop awareness of the needs of mother and child. Environment is important—that means comfort, space, colours, aesthetics, atmosphere. Relaxation is important. That means learning to know the things which make you tense and then avoiding them or developing a routine for alleviating your own tension— whether it be caused by certain people; the fact that you live in an area where trucks and lorries come belting down the road at break-neck speed and screech to a halt at the traffic lights below your window; the fact that your job requires you to stand waiting endlessly for buses that never come; your mother telling you about all the things she did while expecting you, that you don't do while expecting your child; your best friend flirting with your old man because she can nip around in skin-tight jeans while you waddle in smocks that you'd normally run a mile from, and you can't blame him for finding a neat behind more attractive than a spreading one; maybe the fact that your man isn't around at all; maybe the fact that you'd rather he wasn't, because he's driving you mad with his chauvinist attitude of birth being 'a woman's job', which simply means he has the fun while you do the hard work. Whatever it is that makes you bristle inwardly, you'll find it also makes you tighten your muscles, and that isn't good, unless you know how to let go. Which is where the exercises come in.

Taking care of yourself, your relationships, your space and the vibrations around you while you are pregnant is simply an up-to-date version of the ancient theory that the more relaxed and soothed you are, the calmer and healthier the baby.

I don't think you'll find it hard to rustle up several women expecting babies at the same time as you. Pregnant chicks are birds of a feather that surprisingly often flock together. Whenever I would think to myself, my heavens, I wish pregnancy were not such an isolated business, I'd find that a few hours later, I'd be looking round my own living-room and see two or three balloon bellies cradled by loving fingertips. It is reassuring to know others going through the same changes at the same time. Getting together is not only thera-peutic, because companionship is the best antidote to that feeling of being set apart, but it is also informative, and being with other people ensures that even if you don't have the will power to make yourself do the exercises, you can dragoon someone else into doing them with you.

Bringing men into preparation groups is slightly more complicated. However evolved your man, there is usually an element of threat in any situation which might seem to him to be overpoweringly female, so that preparation groups could seem to him like an exclusive sister-hood getting together to rehearse one of the few natural events he cannot experience directly. The secret to his initiation may lie in your attitude. If you exclude him from the start, he will feel excluded at the finish. If you genuinely want to share this miraculous result of the two of you making love, then he will sense it, and you are halfway to including him in the ultimate act.

You must both want to share the child. This may sound simple, but for many people it is not. Some women guard the exclusivity of this time, either consciously or unconsciously, but the outcome for a man is the same. Some men barely consider the idea of being present for the birth of their child. Babies? Ugh. Nasty small messy creatures. And who wants to see a woman with her legs apart, grunting and groaning? . . . The answer is, men not afraid to love. Men who are curious about life. Men who can dissolve their role-playing, recognize the beauty of a woman's strength at this time and want to be part of it. Men who realize that birth can be shared as equally as sex.

Men have their negative social conditioning towards birth as much as women. Early Christianity and Puritanism decreed it a heinous sin for a man to look upon the genitals of a woman, which is probably why some men prefer to make love in the dark. It is intrinsic to their lives because of their education and the morals of past generations. Just as in such situations it may be up to women to switch on the light making love, so also it may be up to us to switch on the light at birth.

It is true of too many men that they feel, and we allow them to feel, so far removed from the moment of conception that they can only view the passing parade of pregnancy with detachment. If a woman approaches having a child as an event to anticipate, a condition to be proud of, an interesting adventure in which the father plays a fittingly active part, then he is more likely to pay attention. If you find yourself up against a brick wall to begin with, try getting him to realize how important he is to you and his child at this moment. Make sure he doesn't feel that if he joins the group with you, or sessions take place in his own home, he is either emasculating his image or happening upon a coven of witches who will cast spells to catch him in some shadowy aspect of fatherhood forever.

Be practical. Think how he likes to spend his leisure time and then see if you cannot come up with an atmosphere in which he feels at ease. If it is only you and he, there should be few difficulties. Presumably questions of taste and lifestyle have already been ironed out, if you live together. If there are several couples then it should still be possible to come up with a loose formula that will combine the ideas of many and suit all.

It's a good idea to serve soft drinks during a session. One reason is that it provides a break from the heavy work, and encourages people to relate on a lighter, perhaps more intimate, level, which in turn may help break down barriers. The other reason is that limbering up your muscles with physical exercise and practising different levels of breathing for labour is thirsty work. There are few things that make your mouth drier than breathing in through the nose and out through the mouth for concentrated periods of time.

Also do remember to put ashtrays around for the men. Hopefully women will stop smoking during pregnancy. Some go off the sight and smell of cigarettes the minute they conceive. But it certainly isn't true of expectant fathers.

It is also helpful to have at hand certain functional teaching aids, and the following list is one suggested by the National Childbirth Trust in London. If you find it difficult for one reason or another to equip yourself with these things, remember the power of imagination. If you watch a child at play, he transforms an old stick into a flute, a gun or a paintbrush, just as his fancy takes him. You can do the same if you need to make a point, these are just suggestions.

AIDS TO LEARNING

1. A spacious room.
2. Per person: one foam wedge (for putting under your knees when doing exercises or lying in bed, it helps you relax and takes off some of the extra weight), two pillows or cushions, one bolster. In England you can buy bolsters and wedges made from foam rubber and covered in cotton from the National Childbirth Trust. For its address and that of equivalent organizations in the United States, from whom you might be able to purchase, see Appendix III. If the suggestion doesn't appeal or suit, try making them yourselves out of foam and cotton.
3. A plastic facsimile of the pelvis for anatomical instruction. This is helpful in that it indicates the exact size of your pelvis and the baby in relation to you as it grows larger. In England you can order them through Educational and Scientific Plastics, Holmethorpe Avenue, Redhill, Surrey.

4. A birth atlas with which to explain the development of the embryo and the passage of the baby during labour (these can be bought from H. K. Lewis & Co., 136 Gower Street, London, and in the States from: The Maternity Centres Association, 48 East 92nd Street, N.Y. 10028).
5. A doll the size of a newborn baby, twenty inches long with a head circumference of 13¾ inches.
6. Charts from which to direct the breathing practice.

Note: more details on teaching aids and organizations for the promotion of natural childbirth are in Appendix III.

There are certain basic ground rules which should be covered during the course of the eight or so weeks of preparation. Each session should include some time spent on the breathing patterns and the physical toning and relaxation exercises. The amount of time you spend on each should remain flexible if the practice is to help everyone.

Then I would suggest simply taking the subjects I deal with in the following chapters and devoting as much time to a discussion of each as seems to be necessary within your group. Remember that needs and interests will vary from person to person, place to place, group to group, and that the time, space and opportunity to exchange views and compare experiences with one another is a very important part of preparation, as is the imparting of relevant information.

I found that when I tried to commit to paper the lessons I had learned, they fell into natural sequence. . . .

Mind and Body Preparation

INTEGRATION—BREATHING—RELAXATION

The three primary things we need to know for conscious birth are how to integrate mind and body, how to control breathing and, underlying all of this, how to relax. All three require, first and foremost, awareness.

The integration of mind and body helps us centre ourselves while under stress. The ability to focus the mind through conscious controlled breathing and relaxation rests on our acceptance of the mind and body as one complete unit. The mind and the body do not function independently of one another. It helps throughout life, as with relaxation and efficient breathing, to be aware of one's totality. It helps you deal with unexpected pain—with pain that takes you unawares and that you want to resist. You accept what is happening to you, you absorb, you become one with it, and somehow you tide yourself over the fragmentation that comes with resisting extreme stress.

That expression: falling apart. Sometimes I do feel as though I am falling apart. But if I gather myself into one whole, and flow with and through what is happening, then the stress no longer appears as stress, and I am not falling apart, not fractured. Knowing how to centre yourself relieves the worst torture. There is an eye to the hurricane. There is a stillness at the centre of chaos. Everyone has a different way of reaching it. If you know how you can achieve peace when you feel yourself subjected to violence, perhaps if you have already some experience of meditation, for instance, then you are lucky enough to have a tool to help you, if labour should threaten to become unendurable. Again, as with the breathing and relaxation, it is important to practise keeping your mind completely at one with your body, because it needs a certain discipline to reverse that process of fragmentation which can make stress more agonizing than it need be.

To control breathing correctly, we have to realize how we breathe. Most of the time we are completely unaware of the process. How air gets in and out of our lungs is a matter we take so much for granted that most of us never question how well we do it. I for one had no idea how badly I was breathing most of the time until someone showed me how to do a Yoga breathing exercise. It was quite simple really. In order to use your lungs efficiently you should breathe in deeply through the nose and then push out the air again through the mouth with the diaphragm. This ensures the balanced regulation of your whole organism and is crucial in helping you to relax. Breathing for labour is just an extension of this basic idea. In exaggerating the fundamental pattern during practice you learn how relaxing and how efficient it is. Like almost everything else about Naturebirth, conscious controlled breathing is really just common sense.

To relax, we have to know how to avoid tension, and to release it once it is there. This conscious release requires special techniques in which we learn how to single out, feel and control certain muscles, particularly those internal muscles which come into play during labour, but of which few people are aware during the ordinary course of life before giving birth. As with the breathing, practice makes perfect. (Exercises for muscle dissociation, tone, relaxation and breathing technique are all described in Appendix I, with relevant charts and illustrations.)

INTEGRATION

We can start with understanding that mind and body work together. It is this constant interaction which makes us different from other animals. It is this simple fact which gets forgotten in a society which separates the intellect from the physique, treats emotional and physical feelings quite differently. Humanity has managed to split mind and body in a remarkable way. It seems to be the schizophrenic effect of a culture which separates mental from physical health, has one doctor for the mind and another for the body, and that sees no paradox in separating mental from physical awareness.

With Naturebirth, we are moving towards a complete, rounded preparation for birth, which informs body, soul, intellect and instinct of the experience in store and what is needed to prepare for it in the best way. It is based on the understanding that our minds and bodies are meshed like the weave in a tapestry. That is the texture of our existence. The mind is only parted from the body in death.

Try to avoid even using terms which technically separate the mind from the body. Once you start talking about 'mentally this' or 'physically that', or the 'mind does this' and 'the body does that' you have already begun the process of separation. Without thinking you have put the two into separate little bags, and set up the conditions for approaching the mental and physical as independent functions, when in fact they are indivisible.

Pregnancy is a time when we should be most aware of the kind of schism this can create. One of the grave mistakes both men and women make is to imagine that the physical upheavals, the hormone changes, weight changes, changes in blood pressure, that a woman undergoes during pregnancy have no effect on her emotions. They are inextricably linked, just as they are in labour. Each psychological change has its physical symptom. This is always true, but is particularly pronounced in pregnancy.

The sooner we comprehend this, the easier it is to understand the importance of integration, which in the end means seeing ourselves clearly. Not seeing ourselves as separate little pieces, each of which is treated like the components of a machine, without allowing for feeling; but being aware of the tangible and the intangible combining into a whole so that each of us is a being complete in itself.

Relaxation can only be achieved by awareness of the unity of mind and body. They must not only work together but be understood to work together. Splitting the two is a form of disintegration. We are aiming to experience birth through complete integration.

Unfortunately in many places we are encouraged either to blank out the experience of having a baby completely, to relinquish our conscious hold of the event, because it would be too tough to handle, or we are urged to experience it on a split level. Split-level birth is the one that walks the middle path. You are offered sedation rather than anaesthesia. The mind dulled by analgesics while the body is still subject to uncontrollable, although dimmed, feeling. Contractions don't stop if you take painkillers; but your ability to control, or take an active part in your labour, is inevitably hampered. The alternative split is when the body is partially anaesthetized, with a regional anaesthetic in the base of the spine, but the mind is still alert. Neither could be called an integrated experience.

I thought I knew what was meant by total integration before I went through a conscious birth. Now I know that I understood it only in the head. And there's the rub! One of the greatest obstacles to feeling is intellect. You dissect, you analyse, you objectify—and then suddenly you've lost it—that elusive something you were trying to pin down has just slipped away, like trying to lasso the wind or hold snowflakes in your hand. Once you try to define your life experiences by mentally standing outside them as they happen, you splinter yourself and deny the spirit.

Yet to accept this, we may have to change our viewpoint; reverse the conditioning that sends us to a physician to cure migraine and to a psychiatrist to treat anxiety, and seldom points out that the two could be linked. No matter how free we try to be to live our own lives according to our own standards, most of us are still irrationally attached to behaviour patterns laid down by our antecedents. Social prejudice influences most of us. We need courage, curiosity and enthusiasm to explore the meaning of freedom, and to be free to experience extreme feelings on levels with which we are not familiar. Birth was a breakthrough for me. I am not so afraid of feeling, or of showing my feelings since going through conscious birth.

I think one of the fears in a woman who has never had children, is the thought that having a baby will be an overwhelming effort, demanding the kind of energy she has never had to contribute before. In fact, giving that energy and meeting that demand does not have to be frightening, it can be exhilarating. Whether or not you find it so, will depend on your approach. The same with women, like me, who have once experienced childbirth as a negative encounter with the natural forces. The remembered fear is of the magnitude of the experience, such depths of emotion linked to such powerful physical sensation. If you aren't prepared for it, if you don't know how to centre yourself, you get knocked off balance, you disintegrate and the thing you reach for is obliteration from fear and pain. When your mind and body are being hurtled into another sense of reality, another dimension, by experience as total as orgasm or birth, the delineations between conscious and subconscious should go, the physical, feeling self, and the self which intellectually appraises sensation should be one. The ego should no longer stand in the way. There are no lines to be drawn. We have to be whole, integrated beings. If we are ready to accept that, then we are ready for feeling birth.

BREATHING

There are particular advantages to knowing a pattern of conscious controlled breathing to use during the different levels of labour contractions. For one thing, being able to breathe efficiently means the baby is getting an adequate amount of oxygen during the cathartic and strenuous process of getting out into the world. It also means that you yourself are getting a good supply, and having a breathing pattern helps you by providing something positive to do during contractions.

The principle is based on the fact that breathing supplies vital oxygen to the muscles which are directly involved with the uterus while it is contracting during labour, and so helps those muscles work efficiently. Breathing correctly also gets rid of the air in your

lungs that has already been used. The exercises, which are for
different levels of breathing, show how taking shallower and
shallower amounts of air into your lungs as contractions get longer
and stronger with the progress of labour, helps you to relax completely and the uterus to do its work.

There are four levels of controlled breathing to learn for the first
stage of labour and three special techniques to remember: for the
times when you want to push, but can't; when you do need to push
and utilize your contractions; and for the delivery of the baby.

You start the practice with the deepest level of breathing, suitable
for the mild contractions of early labour. You take in a deep breath,
and then blow out deliberately through your mouth. As labour
progresses the contractions of the uterus become longer and stronger
and so your breathing becomes more shallow. More of the muscles
of your stomach are involved in contractions as they become
stronger. You have to control your breathing so that you are using
only the upper chest muscles, so freeing the lower muscles to work
with the contracting uterus and help your baby on his way through
the birth canal.

I found that the technique described in the back of the book
really works for me. Since I have tested and proved it myself, and
know many other women who have, this is why you will find it in
the Appendix. It is more structured than some teachers suggest. But
I found it useful to know that having used one level, I still had three
more levels to go to when having to deal with stronger contractions.
Different people will offer different methods, and undoubtedly each
has its points. What is important is that you learn something beforehand which helps you relax, so that you have a pattern of breathing
levels within you at the start of labour, which has become, through
practice, so much a part of you that during labour you respond to the
action of the uterus instinctively. It is a relaxation technique which
helps you go to the point where conscious and unconscious signals
blend, and you do not fight involuntary muscle tension with more
tension.

If you get the breathing technique off pat, so that it is second
nature by the time real contractions begin, you won't complicate the
natural process by having to THINK. Learn to concentrate, and
apply yourself to the moment only. It's important to differentiate
between thinking and concentration, because if you think too much,

131

you don't achieve the required effect. Concentration is direction of consciousness and you can remain relaxed throughout.

There are so many things to take in with the first gathering together of a preparation group, that first-level breathing, Level A, will be enough to practise at the beginning. You can go through it several times as it is useful in all sorts of day-to-day stress situations.

Very often women get what are called 'Braxton Hicks' contractions, so called after the Victorian doctor who first described them, especially in the later stages of pregnancy. It means the uterus is already flexing itself in readiness for the job ahead, preparing itself in much the same way as you are preparing yourself. They are sort of mini-contractions, little flutters across your stomach, a brief bunching of muscles that feels like an intense period cramp. It doesn't hurt, just causes a slight discomfort. In actual fact the uterus not only contracts and relaxes during pregnancy and labour, but all through a woman's reproductive life. Apart from pregnancy we feel it most at menstruation because that's when the lining of the uterus is discarded, which, during the preceding three weeks has grown thick and spongy, ready to nourish an embryo should your egg be fertilized. During that time in the life of the womb, when it is empty, it usually only contracts mildly and irregularly. During labour it contracts with intense regularity and that is the difference. If you get bad period cramps and want to relieve the aches they cause, try using this method of relaxation and breathing. You will be surprised how quickly letting your muscles relax and breathing lightly to a rhythmic pattern will ease any kind of physical strain.

At the beginning of pregnancy, when practising the breathing exercises, it seems more like rehearsal for some unimaginable farce than a necessary reality. It's hard to imagine that you will ever be making loud noises and animal grunts, while you're sitting in the sunshine having a cup of tea with friends. And lots of people feel they can't bear to let go that much in front of a room full of people. But like farting and burping, it's all part of our natural function and we shouldn't be afraid or ashamed of it. One of the points of this preparation is that we rid ourselves of as many inhibitions as possible. In labour as in life, an inhibition is a complication. Giving birth is a basic part of our animal nature and the sooner we clear away the cobwebs of our cultured attitudes to ourselves and our bodies, the sooner we simplify. Embarrassment, even shyness, is rooted in the kind of self-conscious fear that will accentuate pain in labour, so we need to transcend it if we can. Groan loudly at the end of each practice contraction. The more you do it before labour the less surprising it will be during labour.

Don't worry if you start yawning—it's partly because you are so relaxed and partly because this often happens when you alter the pattern of your breathing.

The 'mind-prevention' aspect of the technique provides you with a safety valve. The way you breathe is a distraction. Using it you can dissociate from the turbulent activity in your body. If you want to distract yourself as the strongest contractions roll over you, do. Like a meditation technique, this type of breathing gives you a kind of stillness in the eye of the hurricane. By mouthing a song, which you have learned by heart, your breathing becomes as shallow as is humanly possible while still allowing enough oxygen through to you and the baby. It's a bit like whispering, your breath comes only from the top of your diaphragm as though almost all you are using is your throat. . . .

Before going through each of the levels of breathing as they are related to the stages of labour, it is a good idea to get into the most comfortable position for practice. Sit on the floor with your spine and head well supported by pillows—legs wide apart—if you're going to let a baby out of there you can't keep your knees crossed like a nervous virgin all the time. If anyone else but you gets embarrassed when you do that at home, tell them not to be absurd. Or wear trousers all the time. The sooner you get used to flopping your legs apart whenever you can, the easier things will be on the day.

If you can draw upon your method of breathing instinctively, it can act as a kind of surf board to ride the waves of labour. Doing something positive makes the strong contractions seem less interminable, and helps your body refrain from bracing against the natural force of the child making its way down the birth canal.

Now see specific exercises in Appendix I.

RELAXATION

This is the secret of alleviating stress in childbirth. Everything else we learn goes towards this end, since it is this which lessens pain and allows us to play an active part in our own labours. Awareness is vital to understanding relaxation. We have already discussed mind and body integration. Awareness of this inevitable interaction within us starts our whole understanding of Naturebirth. It follows that accepting the truth is intrinsic to this preparation. By this I mean that painting pretty pictures doesn't help us deal with harsh reality. To delude is not to prepare. Giving birth is one of the most extra-ordinary experiences of life. It can be wildly uncomfortable while it lasts. It can be desperately painful. But one's understanding of and response to pain can change. I believe we can control the degree to which the action of the womb during labour affects us. I don't think that any of it, either the preparation or the experience itself, is easy. I have found that nothing that is rewarding in life is easy. The truth and reality of birth is that for most people natural labour is hard work which demands hard practice beforehand. But it is worth it. Giving birth can be one of the most amazing and rewarding experi-ences ever, from which we learn about ourselves, our own strength, weaknesses, reserves, feelings, so also about our men and our children.

In essence the preparation is about learning how to relax under stress; the stress can come from anywhere, from the uterus, from the environment, the mind, the body, conditioning, relationships with the people around you. Preparation feeds you with information to help avoid or alleviate the symptoms of stress. The physical exercises teach you how one set of muscles can be at work while the rest of the body stays loose and easy. The initial relaxation, or dissociation exercise, makes you aware of the different internal muscles in use during labour, how you can control and release them yourself simply by knowing where they are and how they work.

When we contract muscles, we breathe in; when we let go, soften, we breathe out. It is one of those involuntary reflexes Pavlov was talking about. And the out-breath, the softening and the letting go, is the important one to remember. It is really quite impossible to relax completely, if you are not breathing in rhythm with your loosened muscles.

The face shows tension and strain very quickly, even standing in shoes that are too tight can etch wrinkles into your forehead. So be aware of how soft or how tight your face is. If that is relaxed, it's probably true that your whole body is relaxed. If the skin gets taut and the lines deepen, it's a certainty that some other part of your body is being held in extreme tension. If you think of the mouth as an orifice and erogenous zone, closely related to the vagina, then you'll see the sense of keeping both of them soft and mobile. If one is a reflection of the other and the vagina is *the* area of our bodies that we must concentrate on keeping relaxed, then it stands to reason we should keep an eye out for a pursed-up mouth. A tight mouth indicates a tight vagina in the same way that tight shoes give you a headache and a furrowed brow. You just can't separate painful symptoms in one part of the body from their reflection in another part. To see what I mean try screwing up your lips as you would at a sour taste, and then see if your vagina isn't clenched too, in sympathy! When your vagina is soft and open, as in making love, so is your mouth. A good reason for not being scared to make love if you're pregnant and healthy. It warms and relaxes your whole being.

Shoulders are another common tension point to which people pay very little attention. It is worth taking special note now because they do tend to seize up during labour, and, along with eyes and forehead, are most susceptible to strain as well as showing it most. If your forehead starts wrinkling and your shoulders shoot up to hug your jawline, it's the signal for a nudge back into your breathing exercises and out of the panic. When you are in labour, and feel your shoulders tighten, urge your helper to stroke you gently and then relax towards the hand that's massaging you. Now see specific exercises in Appendix I.

Learning how to relax in unfamiliar or hostile surroundings brings us to the relationship between mind and body again. Much of relaxation is connected to mental conditioning. Thanks to our culture, childbirth is still a spectre of horror in the minds of many girls, whether they hear about it as children, or whether they are faced by it on the delivery bed. Sex education has taken much of the damaging mystique out of sex, and thank God for that, but little thought has been given to the de-mystifying of birth, which could so easily begin at school.

Our intuitive knowledge of childbirth and the meaning of that process within ourselves has been submerged in a bog of misconception. To look at it historically, much of the confusion seems to stem, in the case of western nations, from attitudes fostered by the male-dominated Christian religion. The purity of Christ's teaching deteriorated into a dogma promoted by a corrupt hierarchy in the organized Church; the male was enshrined as the dominant sex in society and as a result women relinquished all self-respect, and with it, the sense of their own place in the natural order of the universe. The gloomy predictions of the Bible became law. Women were cursed. Their destiny was childbirth, and childbirth was sorrow and pain and travail. No wonder fear ran rampant. It is an infectious emotion and it breeds in ignorance.

The only way we are going to untangle some of these cobwebs, for the sake of men, women and children, is to inform ourselves of the truth. The process of de-mystification begins, of course, with women. When I was a child the very first thing I learned about being female was that there was something I would have to go through every month called the 'curse'. Admittedly I learned this about menstruation in a convent, and nuns do have a way of mystifying the functions of the body, but I was by no means the only young woman of my generation whose first imprint of female sexuality was the 'curse'. Although my mother purged me of this notion as soon as she knew it had been implanted, the damage was done, the seed was there, and it was directly linked to childbirth: the next step in the curse. Why was childbirth a curse? Because, like menstruation, it was painful, bloody, messy, and only women had to go through it. With this in the back of my mind I approached my first pregnancy and my first labour with trepidation, and was rewarded with a painful, messy, confusing experience. It was only meticulous and sensitive teaching that finally rid me of these deeply ingrained misconceptions and allowed me to experience the full magic of conscious birth.

FEAR AND PAIN

Through understanding ourselves as whole, integrated organisms, it is easier to see the links between fear and pain. We start with fear of pain. And then feeling discomfort, experience fear again, which makes us rigid. Rigidity is the one thing which will make normal contractions more difficult to handle. Muscle tension sharpens the edge of sensation into something more than we are used to, so it becomes frightening. The less we know of the violence of primitive feeling, the more shocking it is. Expelling life from our bodies is the mightiest primitive function we perform. The more hung up we are in the web of polite behaviour and what 'should' and 'should not' be expressed, the more difficult it is to free our natural urges. To hold back those feelings is to hold back their function, and in this way we counter the normal rhythm of infant and maternal life forces as they work together. We have to learn to express our feelings, not to hold things back, not to brace against sensations. Only this way will we be equipped to handle our natural rhythms while we give birth.

To examine fear let us first decide what it is. It is a psychogenic factor which originates in the mind and triggers involuntary physical reaction. It is an emotion which sends impulses to the central nervous system, affecting muscles and glands and causing tension to spread through the body. We *sense* fear. Knowing that we cannot divide the physical from the mental, we know also that there is a tangible physical manifestation of this emotion. Feeling afraid, your muscles clench, you feel sick, you shiver, you sweat, you get prickles up your spine. If you are unprepared for whatever is happening to you, the body's reactions will be taking place before you can pull yourself together to prevent them. You cannot run from the delivery bed, so you panic, and the panic sets up more hysterical tension. You are reacting against labour instead of acting with it.

One of the first to try to analyse pain in childbirth was the English doctor, Grantly Dick-Read. He felt that it could surely be controlled or lessened without massive doses of drugs and obstetric interference. His theory first expressed in the 1930s[1] was that since pain is psychologically oriented, pain in childbirth is basically the result of centuries of brainwashing, and could be relieved in labour by first clearing the distortion of misrepresentation. He wanted giving birth to be a more conscious, spiritual happening for a woman, without her being deprived of the advantages of obstetric medicine. He changed the words 'uterine pain' to 'uterine contraction', encouraged fathers to be present, and suggested exercises during labour contractions that would relax vaginal, skeletal and perineal muscles.

His premise was that fear influences the inner biological rhythms, yet his theories were not taken seriously by the majority of the medical profession; he was prevented from practising in the way he wished under the National Health Service, and finally left England to practise in South Africa. But the idea that labour can be more difficult because fear specifically activates tension makes sense. According to Dick-Read, the upper part of the womb works

1. *Childbirth without Fear*, Grantly Dick-Read, Dell Publishing, U.S.A., Heinemann, London, 1942.

against the lower part, setting up violent resistance between the two, so that a natural function becomes an excruciating and abnormal condition. If there were no fear to trigger the lower muscles of the uterus into closing against the opening of the cervix, in effect trying to halt the process which is causing all the fear, there would be less pain.

To get to the root of the syndrome you deal with the fear first. Modern drugs deal only with the symptom of fear—pain. Medicine does not offer fear-killers, only painkillers. It is we who must try and find a way to annihilate fear, and then see if we aren't in a better position to experience birth positively.

Another very good reason for trying to do this is the possibility that excessive fear and pain can have an organically damaging effect on the baby. We have discussed the possible hazards of sedatives and anaesthetics which cross the placenta, and may act as depressants on the child. Dick-Read thought that fear itself, without the administration of drugs, could actually limit the amount of blood being transferred to the baby. Although an unborn child needs less oxygen pressure in the blood supplied to it through the uterus than an adult would, there is a chance that if fear and tension are allowed to build up, they could eventually affect the mother so badly that her infant is deprived of adequate oxygen, which could in turn cause injury to its intricate and fragile organs, particularly the brain.

It was the Russian physiologist Ivan Pavlov, way back in the beginning of this century, who first put forward the idea that responses to stimuli could be either 'conditioned', that is, learned through culture and environment, or 'unconditioned', which meant innate or natural reflexes. He maintained that the 'conditioned' response could be 'unlearned', so that by changing the cultural input of information, the response could also be changed. It was called 'psychoprophylaxis', or literally, 'mental-prevention'. The mind could dissociate from extreme physical sensation, and so feel it less acutely.

Pavlov worked and experimented with dogs, but his interest was in human conditioning. This led the Russians to applying his theories to women in labour, and the first pregnant woman trained to use it gave birth to her baby in 1949. It was brought to the attention of the western world in 1950, when, at a World Congress of Gynaecologists in Paris, it was discussed and demonstrated as a form of conditioned reflex training.

The idea was picked up by a French gynaecologist, Fernand Lamaze. A year later he went to Leningrad to see a delivery in which 'psychoprophylaxis' was being used. He was so impressed to see a woman not only awake for the birth of her child, but apparently enjoying it, that he stayed with her during the six hours of her labour, and then returned to France to adapt the technique for European women to use. The first successful delivery under his care was in 1952. He and another French doctor, Pierre Vellay, continued to develop the idea that a woman's experience of childbirth is affected by her reception of the peculiar and intense sensations of labour. Their movement spread to the United States, and is now called 'Childbirth Without Pain', and the 'Lamaze Education for Child-birth'.

These were vital steps towards women's understanding of the process of pregnancy and birth. Grantly Dick-Read pointed to the chain reaction of fear and pain; psychoprophylaxis enabled women to become overpoweringly involved in something other than the contemplation and assimilation of the 'painful' sensation of contractions by altering their preconceived ideas of birth as fearful and giving them a technique of breathing on which to concentrate. Now we must build on those foundations, so that the way we dispense with anticipation of pain is completely relevant to the conditions of birth today.

We need specific information so that we can unlearn our conditioning. In the last decade, our society has changed radically. The demands, requirements and methods of birth are quite different. The emphasis in birth has moved decisively from woman to doctor, from natural functioning to mechanical device, from the organic to the synthetic. If the medical profession as a whole were more willing to communicate with women giving birth, then it is possible this shift would be less intimidating to pregnant women.

Changes in consciousness and conditioning are urgently needed and difficult to achieve. The cultural conditioning we have to shake off now is that we, as women, are totally helpless in giving birth without medical direction, that men and machines can step in and take control of the job, that we are causing trouble by asking for explanations, that pain and birth are synonymous and only drugs or surgical implements can alter the relationship of one to the other. So healthy women have to repossess confidence in their innate ability to give

139

birth without intervention. By understanding the nature of woman, by knowing ourselves, we can overcome the disorientation of strange surroundings, of fear and anticipation of fear, of men dominating an activity that is most obviously female. This is the education of Naturebirth.

Awareness of the Physiology of Pregnancy

ANATOMY

Knowing something of the order of your internal organs will give you an insight into the miraculous transformations triggered off by conception. School biology classes allow the first (in most cases astonishingly uninspired) glimpse of how the human reproductive system works. If schools used a little more imagination in their presentation of the subject, it is possible that more information would stay in our memories. I know that it was not until I was preparing to have a baby consciously myself that I began to realize the marvellous efficiency of the uterus and how it holds and carries a developing child from the moment of conception to the moment of birth.

Before impregnation, the womb, or uterus, is the size and shape of an upside-down pear lodged in the pelvis, hollow with a thick muscular wall. The narrow part of the pear is the cervix, or neck of the womb. It is about an inch long and stays closed, except in labour, when it opens as the muscles of the main part of the uterus contract. The fat piece of the upside-down pear is the body of the uterus and from the corners of this hang the fallopian tubes. Just below the outer openings of the tubes are the ovaries, the female sex glands, and it is these which expel one egg each month to weave its way down the fallopian tubes in search of male spermatozoa on the way up from the vagina.

The vagina of course is a woman's sexual organ, the tube connecting the uterus to the outside, and opening on the vulva, an erogenous zone, a subtly sensitive area, a part of woman to give and receive pleasure. It is this part of us that is the focal point in labour, so instead of shying away from thinking about and feeling the vulva and vagina, let us understand the part they play in having a baby.

140

The vulva has two outer lips and inside them two thinner lips which at the front enfold the clitoris. They, and especially the clitoris, are exquisitely sensitive to touch. The lips are lubricated whenever necessary by mucus that pours from the vaginal lining and from two glands inside the vulva. You will feel moisture when you are sensually aroused—either in making love—or when having a baby. In the first case the lubrication is for the passage of the penis in the vagina, the second for the passage of the baby's head, when it is supplemented by cervical mucus.

The inside of the vagina is a pale pink tube of muscle like a tunnel, about three to four inches long, leading up to the cervix, or neck of the womb. Vagina and uterus make up the birth canal. The sperm goes up and the baby comes down. When there is nothing inside the womb, the walls of the birth canal touch each other lightly. With something inside they open away from each other like the petals of a flower. Half-open bud during intercourse, full-blown flower for the journey of a baby.

The uterus is one of the largest masses of smooth, involuntary muscle in the human body. Before pregnancy it weighs about two ounces, but by the time the baby is fully formed, it is a two-pound mass of muscle, powerful enough to push the baby's form out of your bony pelvis, through the narrow birth canal, and into the world through the opening of your vagina.

The muscle of the top of the womb runs up and down and criss-cross, so it can, like long strong fingers, stretch and gradually pull open the lower part of the cervix, and the baby's head can move down during labour. Contractions are when you feel those muscle fingers at work.

The walls of the womb, which nourish the egg from cell to baby, are as stretchy as elastic to hold the final six to nine pounds that a baby floating in its life fluid normally weighs. They are lined with a rich membranous tissue which flakes off and is transported out of the body through the vagina each month during menstruation. You can actually feel your womb contracting mildly and irregularly to expel the unwanted lining at the time of the month you get your period. Some people say they have 'cramp' which may help you imagine what contractions are like—very strong, regular cramps—and it is useful to know that controlled breathing helps you relax and eases the discomfort of periods as much as it does contractions.

By the end of pregnancy, usually the fortieth week from conception (average pregnancy is reckoned by doctors to be 280 days from the first day of the last menstrual period, or 266 days from conception), the pear has grown to the size of a marrow (or squash), its walls have stretched a bit and are just a little less than half an inch thick. In the cervix, like a cork in the neck of a bottle, is a plug of mucus which seals off the contents of the womb from outside interference and protects the unborn from infection. The baby floats inside the amniotic sac of waters, a sailor in his own private sea, warmed by a constant temperate climate and shielded from shock.

When it is time for him to face the world, the flow of hormone secretions begins, the plug will come out, the waters will break, the muscles of the womb will contract and the child will make his difficult way from fluid to air. During his nine months in the womb, he has had to survive a variety of natural hazards, and the timing of each stage of his physiological transition from cell to human being is precise and exactly judged; failure to negotiate the hurdles or a breakdown in timing can damage the developing parts of the body and its internal mechanisms. The most dramatic and final hurdle is birth.

FERTILIZATION

Let's start at the beginning of new life. Let's go back to the time of conception that is so beautiful and about which we think so little. To begin to understand the value of life, we should understand the erotic dance which takes place *inside* a woman as she conceives a baby.

The sensuality of our entwined bodies in the act of love is rivalled only by the sensibility of sperm penetrating the ripe egg within. When a man comes inside a woman, his ejaculation pours countless millions of spermatozoa into the vagina, but they have a long long way to go to reach the fallopian tube where the woman's egg moves slowly towards them. Only the strongest sperm will survive.

After intercourse, the spermatozoa swim up through the cervix, or opening of the womb, into the upper part of the uterus to the tubes which hang like arches in front of the ovaries. But the sperm is not used to the acidity of the vagina, its natural environment is alkaline, so like man in space or a baby at birth, it has to deal with strange and mortally dangerous surroundings, it must traverse the opposing current as it swims upward, and then negotiate the mountainous walls of the womb before it achieves its goal.

The phenomenal energy of this minute cell is stashed in the whiplash of its tail, which is ten times longer than its head. Magnified, it looks like a transparent tadpole. Seven hundred million sperm could start the race. Few complete the vaginal route. Those that do are nourished by the man's seminal fluid, and have up to three days in which to search out and fertilize the egg.

The egg itself is like a little crystal ball surrounded by translucent film and a mesh of delicate cells called the follicle. Its growth is stimulated by the pituitary gland at the base of our brains. The follicle expands to the size of a marble before it finally bursts to free the egg for its journey down the fallopian tube to meet its mate. It is carried along by the mucous currents inside us and pushed on its way by thousands of tiny fingers projecting from the tube's contracting wall. The tide which flows for the egg, tugs against the sperm. Where the egg floats, the sperm struggles to live.

When they meet, the male sperms surround the female egg, weaving and bending and throwing themselves against the always mysterious almost unattainable female, eager to pierce her armour, their vitality sending the egg spinning counter-clockwise until a single sperm breaks through, and in the union a chemical change takes place which keeps all other sperm from entering the penetrated egg.

Once the union is accomplished, the egg is cloaked in a protective membrane created by the entrance of her mate and, now fertilized, it begins to divide, splitting first into two cells, then into four. It multiplies as it wends its long way to the uterus, a journey that takes about four days. The individual cells become smaller in size and, until they form a connected tissue, are constantly rearranging themselves like the falling swirling pieces of a kaleidoscope held in place by the pearly elastic covering of the egg. Like a circular craft, the egg travels the interior of the fallopian tube and soon after, it lands in the soft and welcoming bed of the uterine wall which opens up forming a shell-like cavity to receive it. It then becomes a ball of cells, called a blastocyst. The spark of human life has found its home for the period of intense progress that will take place within the next nine months.

This time, from conception to birth, is called gestation. From the first day of the last menstrual period to birth is usually about 280 days—forty weeks, nine calendar months, ten lunar cycles. If you have a regular menstrual cycle with, for instance, periods turning up on the dot of the twenty-eighth day each month, you will be able to date your pregnancy approximately from fourteen days after the first day of your last period. However, some women have a longer cycle than this, it could be five weeks or more. The important thing is to know your own rhythm. It helps you know for yourself when your baby is due. Doctors tend to use only the standard pattern, and often fail to allow for individual irregularities. Some women have bleeding which seems like a period, even after conception. Both factors can confuse the accurate prediction of the date a baby is due. Most women menstruate and ovulate within the twenty-eight-day lunar cycle. In fact the cycle of full moon to new moon covers a period of $28\frac{1}{4}$ days, caused by the complete rotation of the moon around the earth. Scientists have noted that the moon controls the movement of liquids on the earth. In the same way, it may determine woman's menstrual cycle and affect the general balance of liquids in the metabolism.[1]

This lunar influence represents the unconscious, the intuitive, the female, the psychic aspects of life. It would seem that moments of conception may be determined by these indefinable, indestructible energies, further evidence that there is indeed no way to separate the conscious from the unconscious or the mind from the body. Science can describe the miracle of birth, but it cannot explain it. It is still one of the mysteries of the universe, beyond the grasp of human intelligence because we do not know *why* the moon influences liquid, nor how the female body decides which particular ovum

1. Thirty-three thousand births were studied in 1938 by Yamahaki in Japan. He found a significant frequency occurring at the full and new moons (*Astrological Journal*, Vol. IV, No. 3). Meneker, an American gynaecologist, confirmed this from the study of a further half million births in New York hospitals between 1949 and 1957 (*New Scientist*, 7th September, 1967). Dr Eugen Jonas, a Czech psychiatrist, director of the Psychiatric Department of the State Clinic, Nagysurana, studying thousands of cases at the gynaecological clinic in Pozsony, came to the conclusion that 'the ability of a mature woman to conceive tends to occur under exactly that phase of the moon which prevailed when she was born' ('Moon, Conception and Sex of Offspring', by F. Rubin, M.A., supplement to *The Astrological Journal*, Vol. IX, No. 4, 1968).

will ripen each month in the ovary, nor why the body sometimes breaks routine so that there can be no hard and fast rule for likely times of conception.

All we can tell is that fertilization usually takes place about fourteen days before the first day of a woman's next expected menstrual period, and normally each ovary takes it in turn to release an egg every twenty-eight days. But both ovaries can release an egg at the same moment, and occasionally one ovary sheds two separate eggs at the same moment, which is how non-identical twins are born—two sperm penetrate two eggs at much the same time. Identical twins start life in a single egg and are born when for reasons unknown the egg divides and two embryos instead of one form from the union of one egg and one sperm.

The first nine months after conception is a time of the most rapid growth in our entire lives. Surrounded by the protective shield of the maternal body, the new life doesn't have to do battle with the outside world yet, and can concentrate solely on the struggle to develop and maintain life balance within the womb fluid. As the sperm and egg unite to create one cell, which in turn becomes a million cells, it contains in that moment of union all the inherited traits the child will ever have. Within hours of making love, a woman can hold within her the secret of another human being.

THE DEVELOPMENT OF THE UNBORN CHILD

The sex of the baby is determined by the father. It is just a simple biological fact that it is up to the sperm to decide the sex. At the instant of fusion, the chromosomes carried by the victorious sperm imprint sexual identity on the new life created by union of sperm and egg. It is a fifty-fifty chance, whether your baby will be a boy or a girl.

The fertilized egg has forty-six chromosomes, half contributed by the sperm and the other half by the egg itself. In these lie all the qualities of the being that will be formed in gestation, and all the elements in the child are equally contributed by both parents. The 'beads' on the chromosomes are the genes that transmit from parents to child its particular physical and personality characteristics.

Once the ovum has arrived in the uterus and buried itself into the wall cavity, it begins to form into three layers which will be prototypes of the three main sets of bodily functions. These three primitive layers are called ectoderm, mesoderm and endoderm, and eventually produce respectively the skin, mucous membrane and central nervous system; the blood, muscle, bones and certain organs; and the lungs, digestive tract, pancreas and the liver.

Soon after the fertilized egg starts to divide, some of the cells group together to build an inner honeycomb which will become the fetus, and some form an outer globe around the honeycomb, which will be the amniotic sac (amnion) and the placenta. For nine months, until the baby can eat and breathe for himself, the placenta is the life bridge between mother and child, one linked to the other by the umbilical cord.

Throughout pregnancy, the embryo child floats in the amnion, which is an oval sac filling the uterus and containing a clear liquid, called the amniotic fluid. This sac is really a membrane. A fine but tough, clear skin. The placenta is a fleshy disc anchoring the embryo through the cord, to the lining of the womb. The mother's blood circulates on one side of it, the fetal blood on the other. The two blood circulations are separate and have no direct connection. When it is fully developed, the placenta is like a circular plate about eight inches across, and more than an inch thick. Its innermost membrane is folded into hundreds of thousands of little flaps, the total surface area being an unbelievable, tightly packed, one thousand square feet.

About 10 per cent of the total output of blood pumped by the mother's heart flows past the placenta every minute, and by the end of pregnancy probably about half the output from the fetal heart is flowing past it each minute too. Two arteries and one vein in the umbilical cord connect the fetus to the placenta, and in this way the mother provides enough blood, food, and oxygen to cope with the demands of the growing child, and takes back its waste products. Hormone secretions from the placenta help to trigger changes in your body.

The baby maintains its hold on life through the umbilical cord and the work of the placenta. Your child's heart is pumping blood to and from the placenta through the blood vessels in the cord. It has three large blood vessels—one vein carrying blood with oxygen and nutrients to the baby, and two smaller arteries carrying blood with carbon dioxide and other waste matters from the baby to the placenta. The three are encased in a blue-green gelatinous substance and the whole thing covered by a thin shiny membrane like pearly silk. A girlfriend of mine who had her first baby without any kind of sedative, was so excited by the whole experience, that when she saw the afterbirth, she thought it was one of the most beautiful things she had ever seen. 'It was like a gem,' she says, 'with glowing layers of metallic colours. I wanted to eat it. It seemed a completely natural thing to do.' In some societies women do eat the placenta. Although this could cause diarrhea, it is full of nutritional value which then reaches the baby through milk from the breast. The ritual simply takes the natural process to its ultimate conclusion.

When you hear people talk about 'breaking the waters', this is the lower end of the amniotic sac which usually breaks as the child is ready to be born. In the early stages of labour, it provides a protective cushion for the baby's head, and as the child moves down the birth canal, it breaks to allow the necessary space. The head pushes the membrane until it bursts. Occasionally the membrane is too thick to break of its own accord, and if a doctor thinks this is slowing up labour, he will break it artificially. Sometimes labour is induced in this way.

The umbilical cord is formed in the lining of another sac, called the yolk sac. Very early in the life of the embryo, the yolk sac provides nourishment while the placenta develops. Gradually it becomes absorbed into the stalk that connects embryo and placenta, and that later becomes the umbilical cord. The part of the embryo which is attached to the wall of the womb becomes the placenta, or afterbirth, which we push out after the delivery of the baby.

The baby's most important blood vessels are in the cord which links embryo and placenta. The heart develops very early in the middle layer of the embryo tissue, and the umbilical vessels are connected with it from the start.

Although with routine methods there can be no accurate test of pregnancy until fourteen days after one period has been missed, it is possible now in fact to detect pregnancy ten days after conception. The embryo is recognizable as a small creature by the time it is twenty days old. Hormones secreted in your body help protect the fetus and help the uterus grow. In pregnancy testing, a laboratory is looking for the presence of the hormones secreted by the

147

placenta during pregnancy. If they show up, it means you are pregnant.

By four weeks, the embryo has increased weight thousands of times and is about one-fifth of an inch long, with the foundations of all his organs already there; the placenta has formed and is working, and the baby is floating around in the protective amniotic fluid. By six weeks the teeth are beginning to form, and by twelve he looks like a tiny little human; he even has fingerprints now, and his heart has been beating for some time.

By the time you are three months pregnant, the umbilical cord is now long enough to allow the baby to move around. Babies like turning somersaults and they like to kick, as you'll soon discover. Feeling these first movements of the baby is really exciting. It brings home the reality to you. In first pregnancies it is usually rather further on in the pregnancy than with subsequent children, because the muscles of your stomach are much firmer and tend to hold in the baby more. You may begin to feel the kicking at around four months. It begins as a flutter. A little twitch. Almost like indigestion, and yet not quite. There is nothing quite like the first movements of a baby. It's like a butterfly crossing your skin only you feel it deep inside your guts. Watch for it at night, or in the bath, when you are calm and relaxed enough for him to play.

This is when you really start feeling pregnant. The balance of your hormones has changed completely. The baby is big enough to feel. You simply have to remember during this time, that even though the bump in your belly doesn't appear to be much of a bump, there is another life in there, which definitely affects your mind and body. You will feel more emotional because of the hormone changes. You will get tired more easily because your body is in the process of adjusting to nourishing another life. One of the reasons some people feel nauseous during the earliest stage, 'morning sickness' as it is called, is that before the placenta is properly formed, there might be a shortage of female hormones in the body. But when it is fully formed, around the fourteenth week, there is an increase of progesterone which usually makes you feel better.

You'll find your breasts will begin to swell. In fact this, and feeling very sleepy, and sometimes sick, is one of the early signals that you have conceived. Tenderness and fullness of the breasts make them very sensitive to touch. You become more aware of your breasts and it can be very sexy and nice, if you aren't worried about it. Sometimes your nipples tingle and they usually get a little darker too, more brown than pink, and develop small spots the size of pinheads. These eventually produce tiny drops of lubrication, like grease, to keep the nipples soft and elastic, ready for breast-feeding. By four months you can sometimes squeeze out a little colostrum, the creamy liquid which nourishes the baby before the full flow of the milk comes through the breasts. When you're about five months pregnant you can try squeezing it out in the steamy warmth of the bath, and later in pregnancy you may be rewarded by the odd spurt here and there. It helps you get accustomed to the feeling of sucking on your nipples, and the rush of liquid through them, which can be very strange to begin with.

As the baby grows larger, the desire to pee frequently attacks you, because of extra pressure on the bladder. At first the uterus, or womb, grows only within the pelvis, the bony structure like a cage that's part of your hips and lower abdomen. By the third month, it begins to grow out of the pelvis and up into the abdomen, but until that happens the womb will press against the bladder, when it is full. Later in pregnancy the same effect is caused by the sheer size of the body inside yours.

By five months the baby is about a pound in weight, measures roughly ten inches from head to heel, and the round ball of the womb has changed into a cylindrical shape. This is partly because if it went on getting rounder and rounder and bigger and bigger your waist would have to get impossibly broad. As it is, the waistline does not go on increasing at the same rate as the uterus is growing because the top of the uterus is pushing up towards your chest. The intestines and stomach get pushed up underneath the diaphragm, which is the broad sheet of muscles between your chest and your abdomen, the most crucial set of muscles for breathing correctly, and vital for pushing out the baby at delivery.

Don't be afraid to feel intensely emotional at this time. It is a time of intensity for both of you—the baby growing so fast inside —you growing so fast outside. Some women think that if they display too much emotion, if they sob too deeply or shout too loud, it may disturb the child, or have some harmful effect. I think it's far more likely that by repressing feeling we affect life in the womb.

Repressing anything causes tension. It could be very distressing to a baby if you hold your feelings in on a tight rein. Then your disturbance is unrelieved. Anxiety makes you clench muscles that should be relaxed, keeps you tight when it is better for you to be loose. Laugh and cry and let out anger as you feel it. Better let it out, than let it fester. Blocking you and blocking him is setting up a chain reaction neither of you need.

By the sixth month, the baby's body is covered in a white creamy substance which is called the vernix. It nourishes, protects and lubricates the skin until after birth. After he is born, you'll see that he is covered in it, mostly the head. It helps him slide more easily down the birth canal and reduces friction.

After seven months the head is usually facing downwards towards the pelvis and his feet upwards towards your chest. That is why a hefty kick from the inside feels as though it gets you on the underside of the breastbone or ribcage, and if you have got a large strong baby in there, it can really hurt. The child will be fully developed by now, but not really ready to be born, although children born at this stage certainly do survive.

So at seven months a fetus could actually live outside you, with extreme care and protection, but has not completed the natural cycle of life within you. If you could see inside at this point, the baby would probably look crinkled and wrinkled and old, the skin still bumpy like a walnut. Although all limbs and organs are completely formed, resistance to infection is low, the body is still small and weak and the temperature-regulating mechanism is not properly developed, neither are the sucking reflexes so vital to keeping a child alive during those first few months in the world.

Just a few weeks before the baby is born, the head drops into the pelvis. It is called 'engaging', and you will see that it really alters your silhouette, so get someone else to watch out for it; your man may notice the change sooner than you feel it. Expect to feel a bit lighter when it happens. You can breathe more easily when the baby isn't pushing so hard under your diaphragm, and you can move more lightly when it isn't centred like a melon in the middle of your stomach.

When he is ready to go, he will weigh roughly seven pounds, although of course this varies with all babies, and measure about fourteen inches—perhaps twenty if stretched out. It is now believed that when he's ready to move on, the baby's pituitary gland secretes a hormone which stimulates the fetal adrenal gland to produce a steroid hormone which acts through the placenta, stimulating the muscles of your uterus and starting the contractions which lead to birth as well as preparing the child's own lungs for breathing.[1]

Looking After Yourself . . . Ideas for Mothers

What are you wearing right now? I hope it is cotton underwear, no girdle, well-balanced shoes—or none at all—and loose dresses.

Cotton is the best kind of underwear when you are pregnant because it is a naturally absorbent material. And you do sweat more than usual, when you are expecting a baby. Synthetic materials like nylon or acrilan do not absorb and breathe in the same way as natural fibres do. You will find that you feel warm even in light clothes and on cool days. This is because the baby gives off its own heat which has to be dissipated through your skin.

If you have vaginal secretion, and most women do during pregnancy, then it is an even better idea to wear cotton pants. Anything else gets smelly and uncomfortable. Tight clothes under or over are a bad idea as they cut off circulation, leave marks and get you more hot and bothered than you need be. A tight waistband can also give you indigestion or backache.

Leave off corsets or girdles, they do not give your tummy muscles a chance to work, although the old school of thought had it that you needed support for carrying the weight of the baby. I have never worn one during a pregnancy, even up until the last day, and I have a flat stomach with no marks. My feelings are that if you have got a good strong piece of elastic there to lean on, your muscles are going to go right ahead and lean. A girdle might make you look slimmer in silhouette for a while, but it is not doing you or your squashed-up baby much good. If muscles support themselves, they keep tone.

I can't help but agree with the Dean of the British College of Naturopathy and Osteopathy who said: 'Women should do themselves a good turn and throw their pantie girdles, roll-ons and bone corsets on the bonfire!'

Women's lib added bras to that adage, but unfortunately and

1. Dawes, G. S.: *The Hazards of Birth*, p. 135 from the Science Journal *Human Reproduction*, London, 1971.

much to my own dismay, because I hate wearing them, bras should be worn in the later stages of pregnancy when your breasts become much heavier than usual and there is no muscle to support them so the tissues stretch.

A woman should be properly fitted for a maternity bra at about the seventh month of pregnancy—this will vary from individual to individual as some women become much larger than others. You should go to an organization like the National Childbirth Trust, if you live in England, or the American Society for Psychoprophylaxis and Obstetrics in the United States, or a shop that specializes in maternity wear. It needs someone skilled in the ways of pregnant bosoms to fit a bra correctly. Normal ones are really no good after the seventh month because they do not take into account the fact that your breasts are swelling by the day, or that afterwards you may want to feed your baby and need something which undoes in the front to save you endless groping around.

In fact, if you do intend to breastfeed, it is a good idea to get a nursing bra before you have the baby. Even though they do cover quite a considerable area of skin and most of them look as though they were designed in the Dark Ages, they are specially adjusted to cope with the abnormally heavy weight they will carry. Make sure the straps don't cut into your shoulders, because that can be very uncomfortable. And try to get used to the weird shapes they weld your bosom into. Some experts swear that if you don't wear them, you'll end up with swinging pendulous boobs of the stretch-striped variety, and even if this is an exaggeration, breasts do need stitched cotton support and separation to help with the extra load.

When I was eight months' pregnant, it was suggested I should wear one at night, disguising it with a frivolous chiffon nightdress, but I couldn't go that far. I just massaged my breasts with almond oil as often as it was within my power to remember; especially just before my evening bath, when the warmth and steam open up pores and invites the oil to seep in smoothly.

A bath every night will refresh and relax you. It's a good calm place to practise your internal exercises for the pelvic floor, or even the first levels of breathing.[1] Washing the day from your skin can be like buying a new dress. You get a lift. All those dusty experiences sitting on your skin are like a constant reminder of activity. But don't

1. See Appendix I.

overdo the soaping, it makes your skin very dry when you should be putting as much oil into it as possible. It is a good idea to put a few drops into your bath. It will have much the same effect as rubbing it into your skin afterwards. Although it will leave the bath messier, your skin will be free of excess oil.

Using cocoa butter, lanolin or almond, coconut or olive oil to lubricate your skin may help to prevent stretch marks, though even this precaution doesn't always work. Stretch marks on some part of your body are the almost invariable beauty hazard of pregnancy. Your breasts get fuller, your stomach gets enormous, your hips become rounded, and most women retain some extra fluid. When all this weight slides away after the baby is born, it inevitably affects the skin. The girth of the average woman's abdomen is supposed to reach about forty inches in normal pregnancy. That means the average woman's waistline will be stretching to nearly double its normal size. Stretch marks are the direct accompaniment of excessive weight gain and are especially liable to happen in twin pregnancies or when the body is holding too much water. Once they have come, they never completely disappear, but marks on breasts get pale soon after delivery. They eventually become silvery and almost invisible. On the stomach, thighs or buttocks they never really go, unless you get so upset that you go to a plastic surgeon, to see what he can do.

This happens because the skin has scarred. When its elasticity is impaired the skin becomes thinner. Blood vessels dilate and, later on, become bluish. Then after pregnancy, when all the extra strain has gone, they have less and less colour. There are some very expensive, very pure creams and lotions put on the market by various cosmetic houses, especially blended for the prevention of skin marks in pregnancy. However, I personally believe the secret is not in the sound of the label but in your remembering to take care before the birth. Olive oil, almond oil or baby oil will do just as well.

I think you really need to start preparing your breasts as soon as you know you are pregnant. Oiling them regularly will help to make your nipples soft, so preparing them for the time when the baby is ready to suck as well as warding off marks. If you do it when you are in the bath, put a saucer of oil beside you, dip your fingers in, and then cup your breast in your hand. Massage the whole breast with your fingers, starting from high up and moving downwards towards the tip of the nipple. When the baby sucks he takes the whole nipple into his mouth, not just the tip. He gets the nipple right into the back of his mouth, and then pulls. If you squeeze down gently three or four times every day, it will prepare you for the feeling.

Your balance changes during pregnancy, quite literally, all that extra weight in front makes you walk differently—and so you should. The best thing to do is tuck in your buttocks and wear sensible shoes. Now I know 'sensible' shoes sounds like being told what to wear at boarding-school, but I don't mean hideously sensible shoes, I just mean—again—get back as close to nature as you can, and if you don't happen to live in an idyllic sunplace where bare feet can skim safely over sand and summer grass, then find some kind of footwear that approximates the balance you find on your own two feet. Never wear shoes that have spindly heels or the chunky pop build that takes you inches above your normal height. Try to avoid boots, particularly rubber boots, because they really sap your energy. Ballet slippers are ideal for some. Light, comfortable, pretty, lots of different colours to go with anything from jeans to slippery satin. Sandals without heels are great in the warm months, because your feet need air, ventilation, a way to 'breathe' through all the exertion they endure supporting your extra heaviness. They get hot and sticky and sometimes your ankles swell. If you do swell, fling off your footgear. Leap onto the bed. Pile books under the end of it, or pillows on the top, so your feet are higher than the rest of you, and then take an hour off to read, or sleep, or watch television or do whatever takes your peaceful fancy.

Rest is really very important. Don't shrug it off, particularly in the early part of pregnancy when you don't see the bulge, so you sometimes forget you're pregnant. That was always my failing, so I know it well. And it's easy but silly to talk yourself into thinking that you are the only person around who can possibly do all the things that have to be done, from cooking to dusting to answering the telephone to changing nappies to writing letters and doing the shopping and driving the car and feeding the cat. It's nonsense. If you absolutely do *not* do those things, someone else is going to get hungry, going to get tired of smelly babies and ringing telephones and wailing cats, and do something about the situation. The other trap I used to fall into is the feeling that you must stay up late, because that is the only time you seem to have left for being with your man—or for being social. Even if you are working, spare your legs, back, brain—make sure they are well rested. Careful organization of your time should not make this impossible. There are some things you have to give up . . . or at least cut down.

Any work takes an extra toll of your entire system when you are pregnant even though it may not feel like it in those first few months. You know you're really pregnant when the urine test comes back positive, but often you don't feel you're pregnant till it shows. Overdoing things in the first half of pregnancy could result in a miscarriage or aggravate high blood pressure, one of the signs of toxemia. There's a great deal of difference between getting out in the fresh air for a good brisk walk, and carting boxes full of shopping from the supermarket, bags full of laundry from the laundromat, arms full of children from nursery school, loads of papers from the office.

Ideally you should be getting eight hours sleep a night, two hours in the afternoon and not lifting anything heavy. We don't live in an ideal world, so you will probably have to settle for a little less sleep than this, and *no* heavy weights. Putting your feet up for half an hour each afternoon should help a great deal, if, like most women I know, your routine doesn't allow all the time you would like in bed.

Finding yourself pregnant doesn't immediately rule out exercise. Swimming is particularly good for you, because it exercises so many muscles, and your weight has the water to support it. It's very relaxing and does no harm. The only thing to avoid is very cold water, as pregnancy makes you prone to cramp. Diving from the side of a pool is all right, but from any height is dangerous. In the same way, acrobatics are bad for you but dancing is fine. It's those extremes you have to watch out for.

Riding a horse, for instance, is an extreme. Not only are you astride a large animal, but it is usually moving at fair speed with a far from lilting movement. Riding is never without risk of a heavy fall, so any outing could end in serious injury or miscarriage. If you have a bicycle, instead of a four-legged creature to transport you, progress will be smoother until the second half of pregnancy. Then your ability to balance is affected again, and you may find it difficult to stay atop the two wheels even if you have been on a bike since the age of four. Besides, it's quite a conjuring trick to manoeuvre your stomach and the bike, so plan on using the machine carefully, and then only until the sixth month.

The change in your balancing act will also affect your aptitude for ski-ing, both snow and water, but particularly snow, since you have nothing beyond yourself to hang onto. Avoid deep-sea diving like the plague when you've got a baby inside you. The pressure changes are quite marked and could cause miscarriage or premature labour. The same is true for flying small aircraft—sudden increases in altitude alter intra-abdominal pressure. When an aeroplane is not properly pressurized, some women have the feeling they are going to blow up.

Try to avoid travelling long distances by any kind of transport, especially jet. Travelling is very tiring, and can be jolting. It imposes undue strain, particularly if you are the driver of a vehicle and have to have all your wits about you for a sustained period of time. Even being a passenger on a train, in a car, hovercraft, boat or plane imposes abnormal restriction on movement and comfort at a time that you want to feel as easy as possible. Most airlines make it a policy to avoid taking women aboard when they are over seven months pregnant, although some make an exception if you can produce a letter of consent from your doctor. High altitudes could provoke early labour, and air crews don't have the equipment which might be necessary nor do they really want the responsibility.

Crossing an appreciable time-difference, as you would travelling from England to America, is even more hazardous and disorienting when you are pregnant than it usually is. Pregnant women seem to be more susceptible to jet-lag than most people, and abnormal circumstances and environment always hold the threat of miscarriage. Best look out, especially around your usual period time in the first four months—and all the time for the last two months. Travel is one of the worst things for stirring up trouble in the womb.

Women whose work is physically demanding are putting themselves under unnecessary strain, especially if they work in the last third of pregnancy. Doctors advise women to give up their jobs around this time, whatever the nature of the occupation. But I can't help thinking that women at home do just as much, if not more work in the running of a household, with or without other children, than most people with desk jobs. There's a lot of physical grind in housework and it is as well to be aware of overdoing that as anything that comes under the heading of 'job'.

See if you can steer clear of standing on your flat feet for too many hours in one day. It's so easy to get varicose veins from standing, or from bad posture and weight distribution, and once they have arrived, they are usually there to stay, unless you want to let yourself in for surgery. There are strong elastic stockings you can wear, if you have a hint of a varicose vein clouding your skin. But the best thing is to think about all the things you do during the day that involve standing up, and then see if there isn't some way you can arrange seating for yourself while you have to be doing these things. Always ask people to let you sit down in the bus or subway. Do not queue unless you absolutely have to, you could catch the movie at a later date, you can put off your appointment to next week if it means standing for hours to make it today, or you could splurge your pocket money on a cab if it means the health and happiness of you and your babe in the long run. If you spend much time in the kitchen it really isn't difficult to find a stool to perch on rather than stand endlessly swilling soap suds in the sink; or you could push a chair up to the chopping block while you prepare the fruit, bake the bread or slice the vegetables. And whenever you can, sit with your feet up. With most of these things it's just a question of *thinking* about them, and then remembering to *do* something. After that, all you need is imagination, common sense and perseverance.

How often and how much you make love during pregnancy is something the two of you will have to work out. Sex appeals to women in varying degrees when they are pregnant, and your appetite can go through many changes with the hormone differences in your body. Some women are lucky enough to find it a time of high sensuality—and I must say it did not diminish my ardour at all and there's nothing nicer than making love with the roundness of your love baby between you. But others go right off sex at the beginning, usually when assailed by the early morning nausea syndrome, in which case it's tough luck on the old man, but not worth pushing or you'll go off it altogether. Also, there is no knowing how often your feelings may change during one pregnancy. When you first find that you are pregnant, you may feel you don't want to be touched, but when the surprise wears off, the wish for sensual contact may rise again.

The first thing to remember, as much in sex as in any area of your life directly affected by the pregnancy, you need to treat yourself and be treated with special sensitivity. The slightest movement can turn you on, the slightest blunder can turn you off. Being

157

close to each other in day-to-day living through pregnancy is likely to carry through into love-making. I believe that if you both want to make love, it can do you nothing but good. A sensation so positive, and ultimately relaxing, releases tension and bathes you in a sense of well-being. It is hard for me to believe that would not be sensed by the baby, but medical opinion is divided in the matter, so advice tends to vary.

Some doctors suggest avoiding making love at the times your period is due, during the first four months of pregnancy. As with everything else, your own particular case will need its own particular attention, and your G.P. is the best person to talk to as he is the one most likely to know your medical history.

Clearly, orgasm affects the uterus, and if it happens at the time in your menstrual cycle when the uterus is usually discarding its lining instead of nourishing a fetus, your internal mechanism will be aware of disturbance, and that is when there is the highest risk of miscarriage, or premature labour.

Find ways of making love that do not exert too much pressure on you or your baby. Now is as good a time to experiment as any, and the more unorthodox ways of making love give just as much excitement and pleasure. There is really no such thing as an aggressive role in sex, if you are acting with love, but by a woman taking the initiative she can avoid the man's direct weight on her and the baby. Try positions that do not involve him lying on top of you.

After the baby is born it is usually advised to wait about six weeks before intercourse, because it takes that long for your insides to get back into shape. If you are worried about another possible pregnancy, and do not want an immediate follow on, then my advice is to wait the six weeks till you have your routine appointment with a family planning specialist, or your gynaecologist. The two or three months following the birth of the baby seem to be some of the most fertile in a woman's life, and it is possible to conceive even before you have your first menstrual period—usually about six weeks after birth. Many hold that breastfeeding is likely to be contraceptive, but this is in no way reliable, and you would be foolish not to take other precautions.

Some doctors prefer not to fit you for contraceptives or put you on the pill till the six week post-natal period is over. The cervix would not be quite its normal size for fitting the accurate-size coil or cap. But you may find that you are so glad to be home, to be slim, to be mobile again, that you are dying to show this delight and affection sexually. Lots of people do make love just after having babies, of course. If you really get the urge, not much will stop you. In that case your man could use a sheath, or there's a contraceptive foam you can use which is about 90 per cent safe, and doesn't harm your tender internal organs.

However, do be prepared for blood loss to continue for some time after the baby is born, even though your sensuality may be undiminished.

The best thing, before and after birth, is to talk out what you both feel and try not to feel guilty or inadequate about whatever course you take. You can have fun together, whether you are making love or not. But that physical touch does strengthen closeness and reassure the shyest woman that pregnancy isn't reducing her entirely to a stomach, and no sex appeal.

Don't forget that the changes in you are physical as well as emotional and psychic. As the baby grows in your womb you need more iron for your blood, more food and more oxygen. Your blood flows closer to the skin surface because the baby is producing so much of his own heat, and the key substance in your blood is something called haemoglobin. This is a pigment by means of which the red cells carry oxygen round the mother's body and to the placenta and fetus. To make the extra haemoglobin necessary to provide a good oxygen supply for the fetus, women need extra iron. You can get this from certain foods (see pp. 198-9) and in tablet form.

As the process of providing new living materials for another being speeds up, so your heart has to work harder and pump more blood around your body—almost a third more per minute than it does normally. Your lungs take on an extra load too. You have to take in more oxygen and expel more carbon dioxide. Some of the extra oxygen goes to the baby's blood and the remainder to you to meet the demands of your own increased metabolism.

The way we breathe then becomes important in terms of getting oxygen into our systems and through to the baby's blood during pregnancy, as well as preparing ourselves to breathe correctly during labour. On a psychic as well as a physical level, I definitely felt more in harmony with the amazing biological activity taking place inside me, knowing that the way I was breathing was not obstructing but rather helping the natural process. We need to be in tune with our bodies and in harmony with the way nature is working for the predestined eternal sequence of events to unfold.

Hints for Helpers

Assistance and companionship during pregnancy and labour are fantastically helpful to a woman. Just being able to talk to someone else about your life and changes is a relief; having someone there to see that you eat properly, rest enough and practise your exercises makes all the difference in the world. These hints are for whoever you have found to support you through your pregnancy and giving birth; whether it is a man or a woman, the same applies to both.

My husband says that when I first became pregnant with his child he did feel left out, although he tried not to. He says it was as though he had to step back from being the centre of my life. He says he sees it happen with most couples.

'It's not that a man is no longer the light of a woman's life, but more that she suddenly has two lights. I guess the male ego finds that a bit hard to take. Having something specific to do, which you know is helping them both, your woman and your unborn child, makes you feel useful instead of useless.'

To him it is bound to be more mysterious, less real, this burgeoning of life in the womb. Remember that he cannot know what it is like to feel exhausted simply from walking up three flights of stairs carrying six months of another life inside you, so do not be impatient when he then expects you to cook the dinner to his schedule, if that is what you normally do. Explain how you feel, tell him you can't —there is no other way that he can know. He won't be able to understand your terrific desire to sleep, for instance, in the early months of pregnancy, and may call you lazy. Tell him there are massive hormone changes taking place in your body that even you do not understand, but have to make allowances for. He may never realize unless you tell him that his paranoid fantasy of your becoming bored with him is in fact fantasy, and the reality is that you just need more rest and less play when you are pregnant.

Going through it together and discussing the changes openly, lessens the chance of either one of you feeling left out. With a little imagination this can be just another step in your romance. It can be the beginning or extension of a re-balancing of the male and female in your relationship, so that each is interchangeable and there are no rigid rules of behaviour.

Birth has become depersonalized. It has moved away from being a family event into being a woman's 'job' that she should shut up and get on with. This is the family's loss. It may even be why there is such a generation gap today and so little communication between parents and children, that children have to call a revolution to get themselves heard. You cannot strengthen a family relationship that isn't there. But you *can* build on a support that has been there since embryo life.

In this century we have become used to women dealing with the children, and skate over men's relationship to their offspring in early years. Apart from the occasional pat on the windy back or kiss on the curly head, thousands of men have no real contact with their children until the child is old enough to reason. By then, of course, it is too late. And the poor men are astonished that their little babies can actually present a concept, cook a meal, ride on a bus, work out a budget for their pocket money so they can catch the first train away from home.

I am not saying it is essential that the man be there. I am saying it is infinitely preferable if he can be. It is absolutely conceivable that a woman should want to have a baby even though she doesn't *know* the father. In which case female companionship may play an even stronger and more vital part during pregnancy. It is also very important that every woman who is expecting a baby learns enough in preparation to be able to have the child entirely by herself, since there is no crystal ball for labour—and any twist of events could leave her on her own.

One of the benefits of husband-assisted deliveries noted by many chiefs of American hospitals' obstetrical departments is the tendency for obstetrical coverage by attending physicians to improve immediately. This was discovered after an enquiry had been made into the practice of delaying birth by anaesthesia or physical restraint until the physician arrives to deliver the infant. This increases the likelihood of brain damage to the infant, and is frowned upon in most places. However, apparently it does still take place occasionally 'in the United States and countries where

Naturebirth

hospital-assigned midwives do not routinely manage the labor and delivery of normal mothers'.[1]

So father can protect both mother and child.

Through sharing the practical preparation for having a baby, John and I learned much about the sharing of our lives in the way of those who would like to see the standardized social distinctions of 'husband' and 'wife', 'mother' and 'father' dissolved. Our liberation from the narrow mores of our elders came about through our children, rather than being inhibited by them—because to us the essence of liberation became freedom from labels and game-playing, patterns imposed by an outside world there seemed little reason to respect beyond one's own experience of life.

John started to experiment with housekeeping and cooking as he saw how silly it was to assume I was any less tired than he after a day's work, any more inclined to be bending over the stove or the sink. The double awareness of me with his child inside me helped him share the practicalities of our life, and accelerate his consideration for the hazards of my condition. Some men might see this as diminishing their masculinity, but my respect for John grew through the pregnancy, and I believe that once a man understands that gentleness is not synonymous with weakness, a great deal of conflict is taken out of our attempts to redefine man and woman in society, and with that, our attempts to find ways for the family to survive become easier.

If we take the precious period of the gestation of our children as the time to focus the unification of our lives, then we can learn to exchange roles without wrenching identities from each other. It prepares us for equal distribution of family responsibilities, and men should never be made to feel less men for doing so. Besides, it is boring to play the same part day after day, or night after night.

There are three kinds of massage which are very effective during labour, and should be practised during pregnancy. They help relieve general tension and aches and pains, not only during labour but also from the earliest months of a pregnancy which may bring unexpected back-aches and tired, swollen feet.

The first is very simple. It is a thigh massage which is invaluable if a woman gets cramps, or feels contractions in her thighs.

1. From *The Cultural Warping of Childbirth*, a Special Report by the International Childbirth Education Association, Vol. II, No. I, pp. 20–21, 1972.

First, gently put your two hands on the woman's raised knee. Then push lightly from the knee, along the thigh, to her hips. Let go. Draw your hands gently back along the thigh to the knee with no pressure at all, then again along the thigh from knee to hip. This stimulates circulation and relieves muscle tension.

The second is slightly more complicated. It is called 'effleurage' and needs a very delicate touch. In fact, it can be done by the woman herself, but is more soothing if applied by someone else. It's good to do during contractions, because it really seems to take the edge of severity off the stronger ones. But if she likes the feeling, either one of you can do it at any time. The plus side of it being done by someone else is that she will feel well cherished and that's always an important aspect.

Powder the skin of her stomach. Lightly put your fingertips on her abdomen. Curve your fingers around in an arc from one side of her pubic bone to the other, around the curled shape of the baby, without completing the circle. It is important to take your fingers off the skin before you complete the circle or it has the opposite of the desired effect, and stimulates instead of soothing.

The third massage is pure common sense. If she has bad backache, or she's in labour and feeling all the contractions in her back instead of her belly or thighs, or that is where she is feeling the tension while she is carrying the child, then firmly knead the base of her spine. Even if she is sitting and not lying on her side during labour, you can always slide a hand between her and the cushions propping her, and find the tender area, where massage becomes like the touch of heaven.

It's good for men to remember that in labour, especially the transition stage, when she wants to push but is told she must not, a woman can suddenly get overtaken by cramps, shivering, indigestion, vomiting, wind erupting from mouth and anus, and extreme chills. She needs extra blankets if she is cold, massage for cramps, but there's nothing to be done about the wind except wait for the baby to be born and make sure she doesn't feel embarrassed—which means you shouldn't feel embarrassed or she'll pick up on it!

If she gets the shakes, try to calm her down and get her to move into the shivering, instead of bracing against it. When a woman starts shaking from head to foot in the middle of labour it can become very tricky to deal with contractions. The most useful thing a helper can do is give an unworried reminder to relax and let the shivers happen, instead of resisting them or being frightened. It is a fairly normal occurrence and doesn't mean anything awful is happening. A verbal reassurance makes it seem less of a crisis.

Medical terminology can be baffling. When the nurses come in periodically to make an internal examination, and say 'she's three fingers dilated' or 'four fingers dilated', they are measuring the cervix and how far it has opened to let the baby's head through. 'Five fingers', or ten centimetres, is full dilation. Then the baby is ready to come out. A helper can act as translator and remind a woman of these things when she is in labour.

Whether the labour assistant is husband, lover, mother or friend, it is important to realize that doesn't mean being a helpless onlooker, or a bit-part player to the mother's leading role. If anyone is cast as the star it's the baby, and there are many things you can do in terms of practical help during this extraordinary trip the baby is making.

Any kind of physical communication makes a woman in labour feel less alone. Just the reassuring touch of a hand is warming. When her lips get dry, smooth Vaseline into them. When her face gets hot and sweaty, spray her with fresh water from an aerosol can. If she needs water but can't drink, let her suck iced water from a natural sponge—and keep it by the bed so you can put the sponge in her mouth whenever she needs it. In the early part of labour, give her spoonfuls of honey, sweet fluids or glucose tablets; this is when she needs to build up her strength. Play games with her—anything from Scrabble to backgammon will do—to take her mind off contractions for as long as possible. Always be aware of what stage in the breathing she has reached, so that you can be there with a reminder if she gets lost.

Some people are squeamish about blood and feel that labour is splattered with it. If it's some kind of an obstacle to you, and you might faint at the crucial moment or something, just try to think about the positive aspects of blood. In most minds, it is associated with death or accident or illness, but in everyone's body it is a vital component of our survival. It acts as a highly efficient internal transport system, is a reliable form of heating, and has its own in-built healing properties. Not much of it is shed during childbirth, and what there is usually comes only at the end, when the baby is born and the afterbirth delivered.

If you are helping a woman through labour, it helps to remember that you may face opposition if you are in a hospital that has a policy against shared labour and delivery. Try to set it up beforehand. Find out whether it is against hospital routine to allow assisted labours, and if necessary, try to change the hospital in favour of one that has more liberal regulations.

A woman about to go into labour today may have fears grounded in that peculiar loneliness of an overpopulated, ill-regulated planet where all she sees wherever she turns is another piece of machinery, another knot of bureaucracy, another unfathomable rule. Try to fathom the rules before labour and, if you have to, bend them during the time of birth. Bringing a new child into the world demands that you take matters into your own hands very often, and you will meet with less resistance if you have prepared the ground before you tread it. In other words, if the doctor delivering the baby knows that a woman wants to have someone with her during labour, whether it is her man, her mother, or a close woman friend, then he is more likely to allow it to happen. If the medical staff know you want a natural birth without drugs, they are more likely to let you try. If you have made it clear that you want the vernix cream left on the baby, want the cord left until it finishes pulsating naturally, and want the baby to be with its mother immediately at birth, it will be less difficult to stand by those perfectly reasonable requests in all the excitement of delivery.

Even though I have had my last two babies as naturally as I could within the confines of hospital walls, it was still difficult under the circumstances in which we live and give birth, to stay in touch with my essential nature and the earth. It really helps to have a hand to hold. The tactics for Naturebirth begin at conception.

Choosing Doctors and Hospitals

In the first six months or until the twenty-eighth week of pregnancy, it is necessary to have medical check-ups only once a month. From then until the thirty-sixth week of the pregnancy, visits to doctor or clinic should be made fortnightly, and from then once a week till the baby is born. This is only a rough guide and likely to vary from country to country, pregnancy to pregnancy.

During this time it is really important for a woman to feel she has a doctor or midwife sympathetic to the way she is dealing with her pregnancy and expected labour. Your doctor should be someone in whom you can confide as well as feel confidence; you should like him—and it is worth taking special care, and moving from someone or somewhere that is unsatisfactory, to a friendlier atmosphere. Unfortunately some members of the medical profession succeed in making those who go to them for whatever treatment they dispense, feel ignorant and therefore insecure. Some doctors and nurses in large hospitals seem particularly prone to wielding the power of authority with a heavy hand. An unprepared pregnant woman is easy prey. She is over-emotional, conditioned to the point of saturation with the idea that she is a secondary being incapable of assessing situations accurately, unable to take responsibility, and she often, unfortunately, feels at home taking orders, due to her own conditioning.

Getting together with several other people for preparation has an added bonus in that couples can exchange tips on doctors and hospitals to save time and anxiety. Urban areas usually have two or three doctors known either for their persuasion towards or against natural birth. This is true also of hospitals. You very soon find them out, if several of you are looking for the same thing.

When looking for a doctor or hospital, either in Europe or the United States, it will be very important to know their general policies on ante-natal care and birth procedures. For instance, both in England and the United States, there are some hospitals that are very much more inclined to induction than others, and some hospitals that state from the beginning they will not allow the father to be present at delivery, while others encourage it.

It helps to have a set of criteria in your own mind before deciding in whose medical care you will put yourself and your child. If you are having your baby privately, try to find out how many babies your gynaecologist delivers a year. Discover his attitude to induction, drugs, epidurals and the presence of the father at the birth. Would either he or his hospital object to your seeking a second or even third opinion on the condition of your pregnancy and your own ability to deal with labour, if you so wished? Don't forget you do have the right to do this, and keep it clear in your own mind that you are looking for a sympathetic human being for guidance at this important time, as much as meticulous medical attention. If you want a home delivery, would he be prepared to deliver you at home, or could he refer you to someone who would?

If you should be a high-risk pregnancy, which means there may be some complications at birth, then make sure to find a hospital that not only has the best facilities in terms of intensive care units, laboratories, supportive services and follow-up clinics, but also has a staff that will be sensitive enough to answer your questions fully and with care.

In London, for instance, there are a handful of teaching hospitals that are renowned for leaning away from mechanical interference in birth, towards providing education in and positive commitment to natural methods of birth and of preparing for and delivering babies. Of these, the Charing Cross Hospital was one of the first in London to encourage women to have their children naturally. The most liberal of these hospitals have preparation classes available and like women to have their men present during labour. They provide their own education in breathing techniques, and are free with information about drugs and the various kinds of mechanical interference which could be used, especially in a sedated labour. The staff often take the trouble to show prospective parents around the hospital, so they are at least familiar with where their child will be born. University College Hospital has the sensible idea of assigning each woman her own special student-guide, who may be there, if possible, for her final check-ups, is present for delivery, and will visit her on the post-natal ward. Unfortunately, many teaching hospitals make little allowance for the fact that a woman might find it disturbing to be peered at and poked by an endless array of unknown students from the first pre-natal clinic to the crowded delivery room. Do check to see whether there is a G.P. Unit anywhere near you (see p. 45).

In the United States now, doctors are becoming more aware of the needs of the family at the time of a child's birth. There are various hospitals, among them the expensive Cedars of Lebanon in California, that specialize in providing room for fathers to stay over with their woman, after being present at the birth of the child.

One of the most advanced attempts at regional natal care in the United States at the time of writing is in Wisconsin. It started in 1968, and was the idea of Dr Stanley Graven, Professor of Pediatrics at the University of Wisconsin Medical School. There is also the

167

Great Plains Organization for Perinatal Care, planning seventeen future centres to be developed in the area.[1]

Yet even in the United States, hospitals that are moving away from the accepted birth procedures of female isolation, mechanization and excessive medication, and moving towards the idea of keeping men with their women for the birth of their children, are few and far between, considering the size of the country and the crying need.

Both in England and the States it is usually easier to find out this kind of information if you are in touch with one of the organizations like the National Childbirth Trust, the American Society for Psychoprophylaxis in Obstetrics, the Lamaze Education for Childbirth or the International Childbirth Education Association.[2] It's their business to have up-to-date news about progressive ante- and post-natal care.

If you live in a large city, you will find that individual hospitals and doctors are publicized, and you have only to scour the newspapers to keep up with medical developments in your area. Journalists and media reporters are always alerted when something new happens in medicine, so just keep watching television and checking local newspapers and magazines. Don't dither for months before getting in touch with a hospital that sounds sympathetic. You need to make contact as early in pregnancy as possible, so that you can begin medical checks, know where you will be for delivery, and have time to change your mind if you find your hospital doesn't suit.

It's important to feel a sense of urgency about finding medical people and a hospital with which you are happy. However much you question the system, it is still vital for you and your baby to have regular medical check-ups. At each visit to your doctor or clinic, you will be weighed, have your blood pressure taken, urine tested and fingers and ankles examined to make sure there is no swelling. It is also usual to take blood tests for anaemia—the haemoglobin content in your blood has to be kept up and you will be given iron tablets if there is any sign of depletion. They will feel your belly, and sometimes give you an internal examination. They can often tell from this monthly examination in which direction the fetus is pointing, whether there is more than one child in the womb, the rate of growth,

1. 'Giving Birth' by Melissa Jones, *Ramparts*, p. 38, September 1974.
2. Addresses for all these groups can be found in Appendix III.

and the regularity of the fetal heartbeat. This is the stage at which we can be alerted for any possible complications, and the doctor will ascertain which standard blood group and which Rhesus blood group we belong to.

It is a good idea to make it clear from the start that you want to know what the hospital, if you are going to a hospital, knows about you, that you know something about you as well as they, and that you are preparing to have your baby as naturally as possible with the close co-operation of the baby's father, your best friend, your sister, or whoever it is you've chosen. But make it clear that you will want someone with you in the delivery room, and that at this stage you are planning to manage without medication. This is a good time to gauge whether your ideas are being met with approval or disdain. If asking pertinent questions, making your own decisions as far as possible on matters like induction and analgesia, and wanting your man to be there for labour and delivery, seem to cause ripples of consternation now, you can be sure they'll be waves of conflict by the time you go into labour. So ask your questions, note the reactions, and then go by what you feel.

Try to ensure maximum harmony with your medical advisers, and strike up a direct relationship with whoever is to be there for your delivery. Find understanding doctors and a comfortable hospital that will not intrude unnecessarily upon the privacy of your birth time. It makes a deal of difference which faces look on you in labour. A woman needs all the assurance, love, and encouragement she can get. She doesn't need hassles, objections, explanations and strangers. If the faces she sees around her do not reflect sturdy companionship and warmth, then neither will she, unless she is stronger than most. Labour relationships need stable foundations.

The best doctors and midwives will be ready for and interested in your barrage of questions. They will acknowledge that you know something about your pregnancy, realize how helpful that can be to them, and allow you the freedom to stand up for your rights and opinions without resentment. This is how it should be, but do remember that whatever your particular circumstances turn out to be, you had the right to choose whether or not you, and your man, would give birth to and succour this child; and you now have the right to choose how you do it. Remember that you probably know as much about you in relation to pregnancy and the fetus in relation to

169

you, as anyone, and that you are going to the medical profession because they are trained to try to define the relation of you and the fetus to mortality.

If you are paying for the private attention of a gynaecologist, you are buying a service. The specialist may be a busy man, may be overloaded with work, but do not let him plead his overwork as an excuse to shut you out from your own birth experience. In England the National Health Service, which enables a woman to have her baby in hospital free, undoubtedly puts a greater strain on its medical staff. Even so it could and should be possible to establish personal contact, if not a direct relationship, with doctors and nurses. It is up to you to convince doctor and hospital of the vital importance of communication. Think about it carefully because the welfare of your newborn baby may be affected by how you deal with the situation.

6

Health

Hazards in Pregnancy

A normally healthy, strong young woman of childbearing age should have little difficulty getting through her pregnancy with little or no interference from doctors and hospitals. However, there are certain exceptions to this general rule which absolutely must be taken into account.

There could be complications in the following groups:

Women over the age of thirty-five.

Women over thirty, who are expecting their first babies.

Women who have had four or more babies.

Women five foot or less in height.

Women who have medical complications like kidney disease, heart disease, tuberculosis, diabetes, gross obesity.

Women who have already had miscarriages.

Women who have already had a Caesarean section.

Women for whom there is a suspected multiple birth.

In these cases you must look after yourself with extreme care, and make sure that you visit a hospital regularly or have a doctor constantly to hand.

Ailments

I think it is necessary to stress here that many of the ailments dealt with in this section are in fact illnesses, and as such should not be treated without medical consultation. I have brought them into focus simply because they are common to pregnancy, and it is as well

171

to be prepared by having some idea what to do when you spot the symptoms. Many potential problems can be avoided if, at the first sign of difficulty, you report the signals to your doctor and take common sense precautions.

INSOMNIA

... is quite usual in the last few weeks of pregnancy, when you may find it difficult to sleep because you are such an awkward shape, or the baby kicks too hard too often. If it starts early in pregnancy and seems to get worse as the pregnancy progresses, it could be a symptom of nervous tension and doctors may prescribe a mild sleeping pill. Try to manage without medication—but if you can't, a calm state of mind is important for you and the baby, so taking something you are sure is safe for the baby may be better than getting more and more exhausted and uptight. Just make sure the doctor is aware you are pregnant so that he gives you the mildest type of tablet, and then never exceed the recommended dose. Or try one of the soothing herb teas suggested in the section on herbal medicine (page 201).

Discomforts and Dangers: doctors report that mothers who suffer from extreme restlessness and inability to sleep during pregnancy tend to be those most susceptible to post-natal depression which can, in severe cases, lead to baby battering.[1]

Treatments: sleeping pills—disadvantages: they may lower your blood pressure, affect the baby as a depressant and taken continually could habituate the fetus. Barbiturates are the strongest and are habit-forming and fatal in overdose (i.e. Seconal, Sodium amytal, Tuinal, Nembutal, Phenobarbitone); non-barbiturates are now more frequently prescribed as they are thought to be less habit-forming and have less harmful interaction with alcohol; both cross the placenta. Psychotherapy is a possible solution in early pregnancy; it's important to find out now, not when it's too late, whether or not you want to have the baby. Suppressed resentment may emerge later in a more violent form. If your sleeplessness is only a question of tossing and turning because there isn't enough room in the bed for you, your old man and the baby—then try moving into a single bed

1. Dame Josephine Barnes, President of the Section of Obstetrics and Gynaecology, Royal Society of Medicine; a lecture at the National Childbirth Trust, London, 3rd November, 1973 on 'Drugs and the Newborn'.

or another room for a while; you will have more space and can read or make yourself tea in the night without worrying about disturbing anyone.

CONSTIPATION

. . . quite often seems to seize up pregnant bowels. You can blame it on your diet, or it can be a nervous reaction to emotional stress. We tighten up in the ass as often as vagina and mouth, without realizing it. If you get used to holding in your emotions, it is reflected in holding back physically and clenching your bowels becomes a difficult habit to undo. The best cure is relaxation. Sit comfortably on the lavatory, breathe out, concentrating carefully on that slow exhalation, and gently release the anal muscles. Then keep a careful eye on your diet. Laxatives are habit-forming if you rely on them for your morning purge and may simply lead back to renewed constipation. Remember: muscle tone is muscle exercise is muscle health. You can handle the problem yourself once you know what to do and are prepared to try.

Discomforts and Dangers: too much straining could lead to uncomfortable hemorrhoids.

Treatments: Diet—make sure you have enough roughage, like whole wheat brown bread and natural cereals (muesli, oats and bran), step up your daily intake of green vegetables (especially spinach), and fruit (especially citrus); relaxation—muscle tone exercise and breathing; consciously let go and soften your back passage when attempting a movement, breathe in, tighten up, breathe out, let go . . . something has to give; pills—laxatives should only be taken on the advice of a doctor and then the stated dose should never be exceeded. There is a chance that excessive purgation may predispose to abortion. Suppositories are better and less habit-forming than oral laxatives.

GERMAN MEASLES

. . . is a deceptively mild-seeming virus, particularly dangerous for the unborn child of women in the first three months of pregnancy. This is one of the rare viruses to cross the placenta and cause direct infection of the fetus, sometimes resulting in serious damage. A sign that you have contracted the disease, which is highly infectious among people who have not had it before, is if you come out in a light, pink rash which disappears within a couple of days. Children usually get it without a temperature, adults may run a slight fever. If you contract the disease *after* the twelfth week in pregnancy abnormalities are less likely to occur in the fetus.

Discomforts and Dangers: if a mother is infected with it during the first twelve weeks of pregnancy, counting from the first day of the last period, it could disorganize the growth of early fetal organs and cause abnormalities like deafness, blindness and congenital heart disease.

Treatment: if you have been in contact with German measles, and have not had it before, there is a special injection called gamma globulin which, if given within ten days of exposure, may prevent the disease from developing. However, it is only fair to say that opinions do conflict as to whether this actually works or not, and you should consult your doctor about it if you feel there is reason to take it as a preventative measure. If girls do not contract the disease while they are children, they should be vaccinated before puberty. In England, vaccination is normally before or at the age of thirteen. (German measles should not be confused with measles, a disease which does not carry the same risk to an unborn child, and against which children are usually vaccinated before they are two.)

VOMITING

. . . usually happens during early pregnancy as a severe form of the commonly experienced feeling of nausea known as 'morning sickness', and disappears after about the third month. In its most extreme and uncontrollable form it used to account for miscarriages and even death during pregnancy for older women. It is said that Charlotte Brontë died from vomiting when she was pregnant at the age of thirty-five. Hospital rest can usually cure it if you get it very badly, but doctors sometimes consider it to be a psychosomatic illness as they find that women who go into hospital for cures, start all over again once they get home and have to face their domestic situation. When you absolutely cannot stop yourself from vomiting, it makes you feel awful, and some women take things like seasickness pills to stop it. Most of these pills are very strong and it is not advisable to take them when you are pregnant, unless specifically prescribed by a doctor who knows you are expecting a child.

174

Discomforts and Dangers: severe vomiting can cause abnormal distress because of the upheaval in your stomach; you should beware of letting it go too far without reporting it to some kind of medical authority because there can be the threat of miscarriage.

Treatment: simple measures are the best, try bed rest and as much calm as possible; the drugs prescribed for vomiting in people who are not pregnant are usually anti-histamines which I myself am reluctant to take during pregnancy as they cross the placenta and have been known to produce pigmentation marks around the eyes of the newborn and occasionally cause jaundice.[1]

ANAEMIA

. . . is common in pregnancy, because the baby needs so much extra iron which has to be provided by the mother. Anaemia is basically a blood disease meaning you do not have enough red blood cells, and/or they don't contain enough haemoglobin which is responsible for transferring oxygen from the lungs to the tissues in the body and, in a pregnant woman, to the placenta, and then to the fetus. It is an important reason to have regular blood checks during pregnancy.

Discomforts and Dangers: it is weakening to your overall health, and tiredness and depression result.

Treatment: lots of rest, fresh air, green vegetables and liver; providing your system with extra iron is vital and you can find that through iron tablets or food; folic acid is also important to your diet because it is a member of the vitamin B group and essential for the manufacture of red blood cells. Make sure you have plenty of vitamins and be aware of the fact that anaemia can be prevented by controlling your weight. The heavier you are, the more blood the body needs, and the greater will be the dilution of blood already there. Excessive dilution of blood leads to anaemia.

KIDNEY AND BLADDER INFECTIONS

. . . must be taken care of immediately. Any delay can lead to trouble in later life. Watch out for the symptoms: very high tempera-

1. Medical Information: Dame Josephine Barnes talking to the National Childbirth Trust, London, 3rd November, 1973 on 'Drugs and the Newborn'.

ture, sometimes going up to 105, frequency, burning sensation when passing urine, pain in the back which may shoot round to the groin.

Discomforts and Dangers: delay can possibly lead to kidney disease in later life. It can be very painful.

Treatment: bland diet; lots of water helps you pee more than usual; regular medical supervision; pills: sulphonamides or certain antibiotics are imperative to eliminate such infections.

HEMORRHOIDS (OR PILES)

. . . are very uncomfortable and unfortunately quite usual in pregnancy. They are swollen, sometimes painful, blood vessels just like varicose veins in your anal passage, caused by unusual pressure; for instance, the baby pressing down on your internal organs in late pregnancy, or straining too hard if you are constipated.

Discomforts and Dangers: no danger to the baby, but extreme discomfort for you if you let them develop; sometimes you can hardly move for sharp splintering sensations in your ass.

Treatment: take the weight off your feet by resting; use a cold compress if they are very bad plus creams and suppositories which you can get either over the counter or with a prescription from your doctor who should in any case be consulted.

MIGRAINE

. . . is a very painful kind of headache which doctors don't yet understand completely. The best advice I received from a gynaecologist was to rest and find as much quiet as possible, because most medications involve either very strong painkillers or tranquillizers, both of which cross the placenta and affect the baby as a depressant. As with all complaints, particularly of a serious disease that could, as in this case, be called psychosomatic, it is essential to get medical advice. I was warned specifically against using ergot—one of the remedies—as a cure during pregnancy, because it acts as a stimulant to the uterus.

Discomforts and Dangers: unexpected and blinding head pains causing extreme exhaustion and sometimes nausea and fainting.

Treatment: bed rest and absolute quiet; report it to your clinic or doctor immediately.

HEARTBURN

. . . is caused by stomach acid and is best alleviated by a sensible diet. That sounds really boring, I know. But it is the most effective thing you can do. Even the good old household standby for an upset stomach or wind, bicarbonate of soda, has now been proved to be bad for you. Sodium retention can lead to oedema (swelling). Swallowing large doses of any other strong alkaline mixture will have the same effect. Apparently, it only relieves the congestion temporarily and quickly, and then generates more acidity. Do not buy medicine for heartburn without professional advice; and make sure to check what is in anything you buy over the counter. Many 'cures' have bicarbonate of soda in them.

Treatment: avoid spicy food, large meals just before going to bed and alcohol. Heartburn is associated with too much weight gain, so avoid too many carbohydrates. A glass of warm milk sipped slowly is often the best relief for the condition. You may find relief at night by propping yourself up on three or four pillows and by avoiding daytime activities that involve bending with your head lower than your chest.

THREAT OF MISCARRIAGE

. . . means that if you are not very careful, you could lose your baby. The signs to watch out for are vaginal bleeding, which can be profuse or just spotting, and abdominal cramps. If any of these symptoms occur, call your doctor immediately and go straight to bed. The surgical answer to threatened miscarriage may be to put a stitch in the neck of the womb. Doctors usually advise not to have this done in the first three months of pregnancy, before the fetus is well established in the womb. The best thing to do is to lie down, put your feet higher than your head, keep warm and still and as relaxed as possible. If bleeding continues, do your utmost to avoid getting out of bed at all, even if it means putting a pot to pee in under the bed. It is reassuring to know that more than 80 per cent of cases of threatened miscarriage are likely to settle down and the pregnancy continue normally.[1] Miscarriages often happen because the fetus is not developing normally.

1. *Everywoman*, Derek Llewellyn Jones, M.D., London, 1975.

Treatment: threatened miscarriage is sometimes treated by providing more of the hormone you lack, progesterone, but there is a possibility that this could produce abnormal genitals in girl children. Oestrogen is another form of hormone that has been used in treatment, but is now known to have harmful effects on the baby. Although vitamins and hormones have for years been the favourite treatment, it is clear that neither progesterone, nor the chemical substitutes for the natural hormone, will avert a miscarriage.[1] Doctors may prescribe sedatives. If bleeding increases and abdominal cramps get very bad, miscarriage is probably inevitable. Try bed rest, calm environment, emotional ease, and avoid taking purgatives, laxatives or making love. The less disturbance you have the better.

VAGINAL DISCHARGE

. . . is a thin white mucous secretion from your vagina. You are much more likely to get discharge while you are pregnant than when you are not. There is nothing peculiar about it. Vaginal glands secrete more during pregnancy. It does not necessarily mean you have an infection. The secretions from the vagina are highly acid and doctors think they may play an important part in helping to keep the vagina as free as possible from infection. As with most of your anatomy, having a baby puts the vagina through changes. Its blood supply gets richer, and, like the cervix, it actually gets larger because the muscles, preparing to be part of the baby's birth process at the end of nine months, become bigger. While this is happening vaginal secretions increase. The amount of discharge varies from woman to woman, but a certain amount is quite normal.

If for any reason you suspect you might have an infection, then ask your doctor for a test. The warning signs are if the discharge becomes excessive, a yellow or greenish colour, smelly, or begins to cause irritation. Tests can be done very quickly and will relieve your mind. The sooner you can be treated the better, if an infection is there.

Part of the reason women get so nervous about infection is that V.D. is harder to trace and more damaging in women than in men, so it is easy to jump to the conclusion that any discharge is worse than it is. In fact, vaginal discharge during pregnancy is quite usual, and usually quite harmless. Glands secrete from inside the vagina

1. *Everywoman* by Derek Llewellyn Jones, p. 234, London, 1975.

before birth as they do during sex. The trouble is we've been brought up to associate wetness in the vagina with being 'dirty', and it's only a short step from there to 'diseased'.

TOXEMIA

. . . is a metabolic imbalance occurring in the mother in pregnancy, the causes of which are as yet unknown. It is also known as pre-eclampsia, and in its most severe degree, as eclampsia. This severe condition occurs during late pregnancy, labour and sometimes after delivery, and can be very dangerous as it can progress to maternal fits, miscarriage, and even death.

The early signs are raised blood pressure, protein in the urine, swelling of the feet, ankles, wrists, hands and even the neck. The disorder itself seldom occurs before the fifth month of pregnancy, and is very often associated with putting on too much weight. Remember that twenty-four pounds is the advised limit to an average woman's weight gain during her entire pregnancy. Salt contributes to fluid retention which in turn contributes to the overweight that accompanies toxemia, so it is a good idea to cut down your salt intake if you are showing any of the above signs. The essential change is when your blood pressure rises, but actually to have the disease, you must have two or more of the signs. Very often the rise in blood pressure is accompanied by oedema (swelling). It is because of high blood pressure that kidneys excrete the protein, albumin, although toxemia is not the only reason for protein being present in the urine during pregnancy.

The women who are most vulnerable to the disease are those having their first, fourth, or subsequent babies, women with hypertension (see following pages), diabetes, kidney disease, twins, or those who have had toxemia in an earlier pregnancy. There is a danger to the mother if the condition develops to the point of eclamptic fits, which last about one minute and can cause loss of consciousness or death, but this hardly ever happens nowadays, particularly when and where women are alerted to the danger signs in early pregnancy. When there is a risk of fits, or when they do occur, a woman will be sedated, probably with the tranquillizing drug, Valium, which is an anti-convulsant. There can also be a danger to the unborn baby, in that toxemia reduces the efficiency of the placenta and the baby can be undernourished, or die in the womb if the case is severe; so too high blood pressure in the mother can affect the baby because it can lead to premature labour, either induced or spontaneous, and the resulting high proportion of small babies are often in danger of dying.

Figures for Britain show that about 7 per cent of women having their first babies and 3 per cent of women having subsequent babies suffer from a degree of toxemia, or pre-eclampsia, a total of about 5 per cent of all pregnant women develop the condition and 10 per cent of their babies fail to survive. One in ten women who have eclampsia, or the most severe form of toxemia, die; one in five of their babies die.[1]

Extraordinarily enough, even the most serious form of this condition could be prevented. Although so little is known of the causes, it is generally agreed that prevention is the best treatment, and that prevention is quite possible if a woman takes heed of the possible signs, so the progress of the disorder is delayed by dealing with the signs as they occur. One or more of the indications may be experienced by a woman who does not in fact develop the disease. But if you find you have two or more of them, do watch out. It is very important to keep a check on your weight gain, blood pressure, and to have regular urine tests. If the disorder occurs and is allowed to go unchecked, blood pressure will rise further, swelling will increase, and more serious symptoms could be headaches, especially across the forehead and above the eyes—which don't respond to any remedies—and blurring of the vision. The usual treatment then would be admission to hospital, bed rest, sedation, with daily blood pressure and urine checks.

Early recognition of the signs is vital to delaying the progress of toxemia. Since the warning indications can appear early in pregnancy, the best thing a woman can do is be aware of them, and aware of the fact that she can help prevent them from becoming more serious by simple methods. A sensible diet, especially one which cuts down salt, can help to avoid or reduce fluid retention, which helps control the weight gain; and plenty of rest can help to control a possible rise in blood pressure. If you remember that when you are pregnant your metabolism is working faster than normally anyway,

1. *Pregnancy*, by Gordon Bourne, F.R.C.S., F.R.C.O.G., pp. 289, 290, London, 1972.

so that carrying a baby inside you is roughly equivalent in effect to walking all the time, night and day, then it makes sense to take specific measures to rest and keep up your strength.

DIABETES

. . . has been a problem in pregnancy for a long time. Until insulin was discovered, very few diabetics even became pregnant, and when they did the pregnancy often ended in miscarriage. The death rate for both mother and child was high. Now life is no longer so threatened so long as control of diabetes is exact, but there is still a tendency for the babies of diabetics to die in the last weeks of pregnancy, although the medical profession is not always sure why. Very often doctors will recommend an early induction or perform a Caesarean section to avoid the dangerous last two or three weeks in the womb.

SYPHILIS

. . . is a severe form of venereal disease. Blood tests during pregnancy will ensure whether or not you have this infection. If you do, it can be a serious danger to the unborn baby, but—so long as the baby is unharmed and the infection is discovered before the twentieth week in pregnancy, after which it crosses the placenta—there is a straightforward antibiotic treatment for it. If no treatment is given, the baby could die in the womb or be born with congenital syphilis.

HYPERTENSION

. . . means that the level of your blood pressure is too high. It is quite possible to suffer from hypertension before you know you are pregnant, and to be unaware of the fact that you have the disease. People suffering from it can feel perfectly well. However, the effect of it can be extremely serious, being related as it is to heart disease, strokes and kidney failure, and can ultimately be fatal. It is also widespread, striking women more than men and black men and women most particularly. Experts estimate that in the United States alone twenty-three million people, about 10 per cent of the population, have it, and between 20 per cent and 30 per cent of the twenty-five million black people of America suffer from it. The mortality rate for white women is 27·1 per 100,000, but the death rate among black women is seventeen times greater than white women.[1]

These are figures to make you sit up and think. Have you had your blood pressure checked regularly? It is vital to know whether you suffer from hypertension, because you will then be ready to deal with the dangers of a further rise in blood pressure so common in middle and later pregnancy. Hypertension tends to reduce the blood supply to the uterus and therefore to the placenta and the baby. As it progresses you may get headaches, or start feeling faint, in which case go immediately to a doctor. Treatment with rest at this point can avert further development quickly and easily.

A bad diet, cigarette-smoking, and overweight, tiredness and tension may all be involved in causing or worsening high blood pressure. High salt intake may also be a contributing factor to high blood pressure as it leads to fluid retention and therefore too much weight gain. It is as well to avoid too much salt all through pregnancy. Most 'convenience' packages, tinned and frozen foods have too much salt in them—added for flavour rather than health.

If you suffer from hypertension, and this is noted in the early stages of pregnancy, you may find that a well-balanced salt-free slimming diet recommended by your doctor will control it, along with plenty of rest and relaxation, and preferably giving up smoking and alcohol. There are various forms of medication, but they can have side-effects, and it is essential to be under regular medical supervision.

Drugs May Be Disorienting and Dangerous

Chemicals affect not only you, but cross the placenta and affect the baby. A drug is a substance which has a pharmacological action on mother and baby.

What we decide to put into our bodies when there is no other life inside us trying to make it out into the world whole and healthy, is entirely our own affair. But in pregnancy, mother and baby have to be considered as one unit, for whatever the mother takes passes into the child in varying degrees. Diet has always been a crucial aspect of pregnancy because unborn babies are affected by malnutrition in the

1. *Essence Magazine*, p. 44, October 1974, Vol. 5, No. 6, 'High Blood Pressure: A Black Epidemic' by Edythe Cudlipp.

mother. Now women have to contend with an even more complex social danger—the abundance of readily available drugs. It is important that the nourishing maternal body and the developing child be kept in the most natural state possible, since we know very little of the long-term effects of the drugs dispensed, or the chemicals in food.

Drugs are tested for toxicity on various species of animals. Since harmful effects on the human fetus from the hypnotic Thalidomide have been recognized (1962) it is clear that toxicity tests must in future include those on pregnant animals. Even with the greatest care in these preliminaries, it is not possible to pronounce a drug absolutely safe. Often years of clinical use pass before toxic effects are reported.[1]

All fetuses are susceptible to drugs, but an embryo cannot ask if its chromosomes will be damaged if it takes L.S.D., cannot read the latest figures on barbiturate poisoning, cannot sluice itself free of too much alcohol by vomiting, indeed cannot tell you to stub out that fourteenth cigarette because it is making him feel weird and shrivelling him up. So it is up to us to think what we are doing to the wombchild, if we reach for a bottle of pills, a decanter of sherry, a packet of fags, a cup of coffee, a joint of grass, a blow of cocaine, a jack of smack, a trip of mescaline or just a nice calming little tranquillizer that couldn't hurt anyone much . . . could it? Thalidomide was a tranquillizer. It stopped women from throwing up, and children from growing up.

We live, unfortunately for us, in a society whose culture and living habits are more than drug-oriented, rather drug-dictated, or drug-soaked. It makes it very difficult to avoid the attendant hazards, even in everyday life, let alone pregnancy. There are now as many different painkillers as there are drops to put in the eye, and it is often said by doctors that their patients don't feel they are being treated if they walk away without a prescription in their hands.

If you go to your local chemist or drugstore to pick up a prescription you have only to glance at the thousand and one pages of the pharmaceutical handbook to get an idea of how many drugs pass through the pharmacist's hands and out into human bodies every day. Drugs which we are now discovering to be risky, sometimes even

1. *Materia Medica Pharmacology and Therapeutics*, p. 16, London, 1963, 32nd edition: A. H. Douthwaite, M.D., F.R.C.P.

fatal, have been given out over the counter for years. Most recent surveys show that man-made chemicals in regular household use, stacked in rows along the supermarket and corner grocery store shelves, are often not only addictive, but can have dire effects on the unsuspecting consumer.

Aspirin, for instance, is one of the most widely used drugs in the world, and considered, obviously, by most families to be harmless, since it is used mostly for the cure of headaches and stomach upsets. However, it has now been recognized that, in excess, it can be dangerous, with a particular tendency to aggravate the sensitive tissues of the stomach. There are five tons of aspirin sold every day, and, because of the way it irritates stomach ulcers and internal bleeding, it is responsible for the loss of some twenty thousand gallons of blood a year, because of internal hemorrhaging.[1]

Aspirin, if taken in large doses by the mother during pregnancy, can provoke a miscarriage and cause hemorrhage or death in the newborn. Other widely used drugs, which admittedly now require prescription, are amphetamines to pep you up and barbiturates to put you to sleep. Currently fifteen million barbiturate prescriptions are issued every year in the U.K., and there have been as many as five million amphetamine prescriptions in one year, although these figures have dropped lately. Both are highly addictive and fatal in overdose, as is aspirin.

Caffeine, nicotine and alcohol, taken in excess, are all under suspicion as being harmful to the fetus.[1] Nicotine is practically rammed down our throats in the shape of cigarettes from the moment we can read, watch television, go to the movies or be present at a normal community social gathering. Yet it is one of the most powerful drugs, along with alcohol, there is. Smokers' babies are known to be born smaller than average, often premature, and nicotine is now widely believed to cause damage to the unborn. The medical advisor to a large circulation woman's magazine in England, Dr Phillip Lawson, has stated that nicotine is one of the most poisonous of all known drugs and acts on the body with the 'rapidity of cyanide'.[2] The nicotine in tobacco smoke affects almost every organ in the body and plays havoc with the central nervous system.

1. *British Medical Journal*, p. 545, 2nd September, 1972.
2. 'Ecology of the Womb', by M. L. Houston, *Expecting Magazine*, Winter 1973–4, U.S.A.

Inhaling tobacco smoke means you are inhaling carbon monoxide, a poisonous gas. Doctors think a high carbon monoxide level in the blood might account for the lower weight of smokers' babies. This anxiety led Sir Keith Joseph, when he was Britain's Minister for Health, to demand that tobacco companies reveal the amount of carbon monoxide inhaled from their brands of cigarette, but so far there has been so little stress on the dangers, particularly to the unborn, that few people realize the seriousness of the problem.

Britain's National Child Development Study, set up in 1958 to follow the growth and maturation of fifteen thousand children born in England, Scotland and Wales, led to the National Children's Bureau being introduced in 1963. The huge amount of facts, gathered on this sample of children, contributed to a report published in 1963 which showed that the death rate of infants born to mothers who had smoked during pregnancy was 26 per cent higher than that of infants born to women who did not smoke. In 1969 a follow-up survey showed that the seven-year-old children of women who had smoked during pregnancy were on average shorter in height and also had more problems at school than the seven-year-old children whose mothers had not smoked while they were pregnant.

EFFECTS ON THE FETUS OF THE FOLLOWING DRUGS ARE:

Nicotine	smaller babies, sometimes wrinkled, sometimes premature.
Alcohol	a degree of intoxication, a baby born to an alcoholic mother would suffer withdrawal.
Caffeine (in coffee) *and Tannic acid* (in tea)	these are mildly addictive stimulants, with diuretic effects to the mother. They cross the placenta, and taken to excess may act as a stimulant on the baby's system.
Marijuana	no evidence of ill-effects to the fetus.
Barbiturate sleeping pills	these cross the placenta and alter the fetal environment, acting as a depressant.
Non-barbiturate sleeping pills	slightly less harmful than barbiturates as they are not so addictive; some doctors would rather not prescribe these during

185

	pregnancy as their effects are less well researched than barbiturates which have been around longer.
Tranquillizers	these might be prescribed in a tense pregnancy, but also cross the placenta with some depressant effect on the fetus.
Lysergic acid Dethylamide (L.S.D., acid)	this, and the following hallucinogenic or psychedelic drugs, should emphatically be avoided, especially in the mid-term of pregnancy—there is possible risk of miscarriage. L.S.D. increases the metabolic rate and alters consciousness in the user, sometimes to the point of extreme disorientation. It has not been proved either physiologically or psychologically harmful, or physically addictive, but some doctors hold the theory that it could cause chromosome damage in the mother and possibly the unborn. There is no conclusive evidence. However, it is common sense to avoid such an extremely strong drug during pregnancy. Since drugs cross the placenta and L.S.D. has sometimes violent physical and psychological effects, there is the ever-present danger of miscarriage.
	Note: this is obviously far too risky a drug to take deliberately during pregnancy, but if you find out you are pregnant and have taken it since the date of conception, tests can be made for suspected abnormalities in the fetus after the sixth week of pregnancy, although it is usually left till between twelve and fourteen weeks.
Peyote (Mexican cactus buttons) *Mescaline* (derived from peyote)	all are strong organic hallucinogenics whose effects increase the maternal heart rate. This can be harmful to the fetus, in that the amount taken is difficult to

186

Psylocybin (derived from the Mexican sacred mushroom)

assess and, as with any sudden change to the system during pregnancy, miscarriage could result.

Amphetamines

these are stimulants which produce dependence in the user. They speed up the mental functioning, reduce appetite and make the body work faster than it should and could similarly affect the baby's heartrate.

Cocaine

an addictive nervous stimulant from the cocoa leaf, medicinally used as a local anaesthetic, especially for the eye and nasal lining; this is a strong stimulant and should be avoided since it can also stimulate the baby's heartrate.

Heroin

a substance obtained from chemical treatment of morphine; a highly addictive narcotic depressant which crosses the placenta and if used regularly can cause the baby to become addicted; causes acute constipation in habitual users who are vulnerable to hepatitis or jaundice, diseases which could also affect the fetus. Heroin addicts are now being treated with a substitute, less euphoric drug called Methadone.

Note: if the mother is taking either drug with regularity they cross the placenta and, both being physiologically addictive, the baby would be born an addict and suffer withdrawal symptoms after birth. If you know you are an addict it would be a good idea to check with your hospital, register with a treatment clinic, and warn the doctor, or medical staff, who will deliver you. Be prepared for the possible eventuality of your baby having to have a transfusion when he is born.

Morphine	strong addictive painkiller derived from the natural source, opium, which has a depressant effect on the baby's system in much the same way as heroin, although it is less strong, weight for weight, in its effect.
Aspirin	can cause stomach ulcers and gastric disorders, large amounts can cause hemorrhage in the newborn, and miscarriage.
Phenacetin	dangerous for the kidneys of the mother and probably of the baby.
Antibiotics	are used for treating chronic infections; all cross the placenta and some should be avoided by expectant mothers as they can cause yellowing in the teeth of the baby. Tetracycline stains the baby's teeth. Streptomycin has been associated with rare cases of deafness in children. Long-acting sulphonamides, given to the mother, can cause jaundice in the infant.
Antihistamines	are usually prescribed to stop vomiting. Be especially careful of which kind you take during pregnancy because they do cross the placenta and may result in jaundice and possible pigmentation marks around the eyes of the newborn. Some have been especially developed for early pregnancy; others are not advised.
Cortisone	is one of a group of steroid hormones used for a variety of purposes, which in large doses can give rise to abnormalities of the fetus and placenta. In particular it can cause cleft lip, and sometimes palate; it can also lead to stillbirth.
Progesterone	is one of the hormones secreted by the ovary, and in pregnancy by the placenta; progesterone treatment is given in cases of hormone deficiency and sometimes for

preventing miscarriage; its synthetic coun-
terpart, progestogen, should be used with
extreme care as female children have shown
signs of genital masculinization (male
children are not affected).

Diet

It is of paramount importance to be aware of your diet. The
things you eat affect the baby and your own metabolism. Your diet
can either cause or prevent overweight, and some doctors believe a
nutritious diet may be a strong factor in the prevention, and even
cure, of maternal toxemia. Eating the right food can obviate the need
for medication. Your body is well designed, not only for carrying a
child, but for warding off disease.

Doctors usually recommend a limit to the amount of weight it is
advisable to gain during pregnancy. This varies from doctor to
doctor. A sensible limit is around twenty-four pounds for the whole
pregnancy, but each of us has a slightly different metabolic rate, and
America's National Research Council now recommends that a pregnant woman should feel free to gain weight as long as it is from eating
nourishing healthy food, and not from gorging cream buns and ice-
cream and potato crisps, none of which have nutritional value, but
all of which put on weight by causing a woman to retain fat and fluid.

Dr Tom Brewer, an obstetrician from California, who is renowned
for his pioneering work in the field of nutrition in pregnancy,
believes that it is entirely possible to prevent metabolic toxemia of
late pregnancy by controlled diet. Since the risk of a degree of
toxemia affects so many pregnant women, it is worth following a few
basic rules of diet, the main features of which are a good supply of
protein and few carbohydrates.

Dr Brewer did four years of research at Jackson Memorial
Hospital in Miami, and produced evidence that toxemia is directly
related to malnutrition, which adversely affects the liver. Liver
dysfunction results in such abnormalities as oedema (pronounced
swelling), and arterial hypertension. The liver makes albumin, and
toxemia patients have what is called 'low serum albumin'. This means
that as the albumin level falls, the water and salt from the blood leak
out into the spaces between cells, creating pathological oedema.

Another function of the liver is to conjugate and excrete through

bile and kidneys the excess female hormones, oestrogen and progesterone, produced in large quantities by the placenta during
pregnancy. When the liver is not working properly, which could be
due to malnutrition, it cannot detoxify, so the hormones are not
eliminated from the body as they should be, and they accumulate
in abnormal quantity, and are potentially toxic. Good nutrition,
particularly an adequate protein intake, helps the pregnant woman
to cope with this. When the liver is functioning well, it produces
special 'binding' proteins which render the excess hormone levels
'metabolically inert'.[1]

Vitamins A and B_3 (Niacin) and C are all necessary for the
synthesis or binding of these hormones.[2] Since oestrogen and
progesterone are in your system throughout pregnancy, the vitamins
needed for their synthesis should be in your diet. There is a particularly risky time around the twelfth or fourteenth week of pregnancy
which is usually around the third missed period when the stimulation
of the hormones shifts from ovary to placenta.[3] Sometimes the
placenta doesn't take over immediately the ovaries cease their
production. This is when there is the greatest risk of miscarriage, and
the greatest need for vitamins A, B and C in the food you eat. So
make sure you are getting fish liver oil for vitamin A; B complex
supplements like yeast, wheat germ and desiccated liver; and vitamin
C in fruit, vegetables and rose hips.

Dr Brewer is violently against the use of drugs to control toxemia.
In an article in the Current Opinion column of *Medical Tribune*
(26th July, 1972) he writes that he blames the 'hard sell' of diuretics
and amphetamines for the lack of emphasis put on nutrition during
pregnancy.

'Some drug firms after 1958 jumped on the bandwagon and began
to promote not only salt diuretics but also amphetamines and
other "appetite depressants" for weight control in human pregnancy.'
He estimates some twenty-two million pregnancies have been treated
by this food-restricted medicated regime since 1958, when drug
companies initiated their promotional campaign for obstetrical use
of diuretics.

1. Dr Charles Lloyd, in *Textbook of Endocrinology*, by W. B. Saunders.
2. Dr Isobel Jennings, in *Vitamins in Endocrine Metabolism*, by Charles C.
Thomas.
3. Dr K. J. Catt, in *An ABC of Endocrinology*, Little Brown & Co.

190

The rate of mothers dying from toxemia per hundred thousand of live births in the United States is 6·2, but it gets as high as 30·2 in Mississippi and 20·3 in South Carolina, the two states with the lowest per capita income where women are least likely to be able to maintain a nutritional diet.

These statistics caused Nicholas J. Eastman, M.D., Professor Emeritus, Department of Obstetrics, Johns Hopkins Hospital, U.S.A., to respond to Brewer's thesis of prevention through nutrition, by admitting: 'This strikes me as very convincing evidence that malnutrition does play an important, possibly the most important, part in the etiology of the toxemias.'[1]

There are figures available for the year 1958 which show that 1,581 women died in the course of 4,203,812 births, and hemorrhage, puerperal infection and toxemia of pregnancy accounted for 75 per cent of these deaths. In the same year stillbirths or neonatal mortality accounted for 175,000 deaths in children. After considerable study relating nutrition to pregnancy it has been concluded that 'over fifty per cent of these deaths could have been prevented with the application of present knowledge'.[2]

Professor Eastman and Professor Hellman, Chairman of the Department of Obstetrics and Gynecology at the State University of New York, point out that obstetrics 'owes much to the science of nutrition and in time will probably owe more, since many disturbances of pregnancy are suspected of being dietary in origin'.[3]

Malnutrition, which is a more serious condition of vitamin deficiency than simply eating unwisely, is now blamed for the death of some thirty thousand babies a year in the United States, and there's little doubt that a poorly nourished mother is likely to give birth to a lower than average weight baby. It looks as though the babies in danger of serious malnutrition might have growth depression and possibly mental retardation. Dr Charles Lowe, formerly Chairman of the American Academy of Pediatrics Nutrition Committee, writes:

1. *Prevention Magazine*, 'Don't Risk Toxemia in Pregnancy', p. 103, January 1972.
2. Eastman, N. J. and Hellman, L. M.: *Williams Obstetrics*, 12th ed., 1961, New York, Appleton-Century-Crofts.
3. *Ibid.*

'An infant so endowed most likely will become a handicapped adult if he survives.'[1]

Another nutritionist, Myron Winick, at Cornell University, U.S.A., points out that:

'If malnutrition occurs during pregnancy or the first six months of life when the brain cells are rapidly dividing, permanent stunting of the brain may occur. If malnutrition occurs after the first six months, a child's learning ability may be seriously reduced. While the second type can be remedied with proper diet, the first type of damage is uncorrectable.'

A woman carrying a child needs full nutrition not only for her own normal metabolic needs and those of the growing baby, but also for handling the abnormal quantities of hormones circulating through her system and for mediating changed body processes which these hormones induce.

High-quality protein foods are meat, fish, fowl, milk and cheese. They provide all the essential amino acids that the body needs to build its own protein molecules. A good diet is common sense.

Natural Medicines

We have considered the effects and possible after-effects of currently available and widely used pharmacological substances for the treatment of particular ailments in pregnancy. If people are curious as to what they could do to help themselves without recourse to chemicals or manufactured drugs, there are alternatives. I draw your attention to homoeopathy and herbal remedies.

HOMOEOPATHY

Homoeopathy is one of the oldest existing forms of medicine, but yet not considered generally as being 'orthodox' in the sense of being 'conventionally approved'. It works on the 'Law of Similars'. It is known as the 'Medicine of Likes'—the pathy of like sickness, because its medicines are used only to cure the exact symptoms they would produce in the healthy. For this reason their dosage is absolutely crucial, and homoeopathic prescriptions are best given under the guidance of a homoeopathic practitioner.

1. Dr Charles Lowe, *Chicago Tribune*, 9th November, 1971.

The physician who most carefully documented his experiments with homoeopathy is Dr Samuel Hahnemann, considered to be one of the great analytical chemists of his day.[1] He was born in 1775 in South-west Germany, and lived until 1843. He said that his work meant learning to deal with facts—'facts simply expressed in the changeless language of Nature'. He believed that medicine should be concerned with cutting out the root of pain, not deadening the symptoms. He found that a child with scarlet fever is consumed by the same hallucinogenic fantasies and rocketing temperatures as someone who has taken the poison belladonna. By dosing the patient with a minute amount of belladonna he found he could release the drug's curative powers and rapidly reduce the fever. By the age of twenty-five, he had established a tradition of medicine which was widely used before all medicine became based on pharmacology. Homoeopathy is enjoying increased popularity as an alternative to technological medicine today.

Homoeopathic medicine during pregnancy stresses awareness that care of the child begins in the uterus, and therefore it is 'essential to guard the mental and physical well-being of the mother if the best possible child is to be born'.[2] It is a medicine which takes into account the overall health picture, allowing for emotional and physical states of being, rather than simply dealing with physical symptoms.

It is always advisable to be under the guidance of a specialist in any form of medicine. In the case of orthodox medicine it would be an orthodox doctor, in the case of herb treatments it would be a medical herbalist, in the case of homoeopathy it would be a homoeopathic doctor. If you want to try some of these remedies, then remember that what I tell you is only a brief guide, to give you some idea of what is available, for what, and why. If you do decide to explore the possibilities, what follows is an indication of the remedies a homoeopathic doctor would prescribe, and gives some clues to self-help if you cannot find a specialist in homoeopathy to help you. I culled my own information and advice, particular to pregnancy, from my doctor, who is both an M.D. (Doctor of Medicine in the

1. *Homoeopathy*, by G. Ruthven Mitchell, L.R.C.P.& S.Edin., L.R.F.P.S.& F.F.Hom., W. H. Allen, London, 1975.
2. *Homoeopathy for Mother and Infant*, Douglas M. Borland, M.B., Ch.B., F.F.Hom., British Homoeopathic Association.

orthodox sense) and a homoeopath, well skilled in the ways and needs of alternative living. It has been checked by the Secretary of the British Homoeopathic Association in London.

The advice in this and the following section about herbs neither cuts out the regular physician nor tub-thumps for doctoring yourself without guidance. It is simply to say that if you are not entirely happy with the existing medical establishment, what it offers in the case of certain conditions and how, there are alternatives.

Constipation is quite usual in pregnancy but not very good for either you or the baby. So eat plenty of green vegetables and fruit, and try *Nux Vomica*, a homoeopathic remedy.

Note: chronic (or extreme) constipation would need special attention, and may take several months to cure.

Diarrhea in early pregnancy is another maternal discomfort which should be watched carefully as it could lead to the toxic matter from the mother adversely affecting the fetus. Do not let diarrhea last longer than two days without treatment. Treat it with *Mercurius*.

German measles is widely known to be very dangerous to the baby if the mother contracts it within the first three months of pregnancy. If you should be exposed to the disease, you would probably be given *Rubella Nosode* by a homoeopathic doctor so that you can quickly begin to build up the body's resistance to the disease.

Hemorrhoids can sometimes blow up, especially towards the end of pregnancy, simply from so much pressure from the baby on your anus. They are little swollen blood vessels or veins which appear in the anal canal like hard bumps and really hurt if you strain your bowels. Use *Aesculus* (horse chestnut) cream and suppositories, or try carrying a conker (horse chestnut) in your pocket! *Witch Hazel* in a homoeopathic potency also helps to cool and soothe the soreness.

Indigestion and wind from over-eating, drinking, or food that is too rich is the perpetual tom-tom of the pregnant native. Try the homoeopathic charcoal *Carbo Veg*, or again *Nux Vomica*—which has to be prescribed by a homoeopathic doctor.

Excessive vomiting if allowed to go on for longer than twenty-four hours can get out of hand and lead to miscarriage or premature birth if not controlled. Try *Ipecacuanha* to control and soothe the uterine spasms which cause vomiting.

Albuminuria is a sign of strain in both mother and child. It is a kidney secretion which shows up in the mother's urine. It indicates insufficient elimination of toxic wastes. Put as little strain as possible on the kidneys by eating only bland foods and drink quantities of liquid to flush out toxic materials. Try *Juniper* as a diuretic, or *Berberis Vulgaris*, or *Solidago* (the plant, Golden Rod). By allowing the mother to eliminate sufficiently, organs like the kidneys tone up. (These last three remedies can either be taken in the form of homoeopathic tinctures or dried herbs.)

Dizzy or fainting spells are usually due either to exhaustion, in which case eat lots and get plenty of sleep and relaxation; or to some kind of mental or emotional disturbance. The above common-sense remedy applies to both conditions, but for the latter homoeopathy suggests *Natrum Muriaticum* for soothing baby blues. It is quite simply salt, in homoeopathic dosage, but it is said to be marvellous for clearing tears, fears, unfounded suspicions, jealousy, and that irrational craving for sympathy that sometimes overwhelms you when you're pregnant. It also helps cure headaches and the anguish from whence the headaches came.

Threatened miscarriage might arise from poor muscle tone in the uterus. Try *Lappa Arctium* (Burdock), which is sometimes called a 'uterine magnet' because it tones up the muscles of the uterus and is used to right a prolapsed womb.

Home Homoeopathy

Here is a suggested standby kit for pregnancy. The medicines listed are those most likely to be needed while you are pregnant and would be useful to have with you. Ask your homoeopathic doctor or chemist if they could be given to you in correct dosage, with explicit directions as to how often they should be taken.

Ipecacuanha	to reduce nausea.
Arnica	the great remedy for any bruised parts; a cure for any kind of bruising and made from an Alpine flower, Arnica is carried everywhere by ski-ers to ease bruised limbs and the trauma of accident; North American Indians in the Rocky Mountains take the same precautions; it is great for improving the condition of mind

and body in crisis and applies particularly to the bumps and bruises which may occur in the less agile days of late pregnancy; taken just before and just after delivery it relieves the birth trauma and helps stop bleeding.

Arsenicum album is excellent if you feel in any way hung-over from too much drink, food, or drugs; solves digestive problems, flatulence, wind and constipation.

Aesculus cream for hemorrhoids.

Phosphorus levels out flash cravings and soothes a sensitive abdomen, also takes away fear and calms the desire to be constantly reassured and caressed;

it builds strong bones in the baby and if you feel indifferent towards those you love or are turned off sex it helps redress the balance;

also relieves the kind of whim-nausea you can get in pregnancy, when just the faintest whiff of a greasy pan or meat going off can make you heave in disgust;

useful to have around if your sense of smell is more delicate in pregnancy.

Caulophyllum (squaw root) is important in any pregnancy kit as it specifically affects the uterus; discovered and used first by the North American Indians, they take it to help towards a quick and easy labour; the Indians chew the root and say that if you take it once a month, in the morning and the evening of the day which begins each month of the pregnancy, and then once a day in the last three weeks of pregnancy, your uterus will be in peak condition for the work it has to do; you can prepare your womb with a sustained course throughout pregnancy if you take it in homoeopathic dosage, but it is essential to check the potency, whether you take it periodically throughout pregnancy or only just before and just after delivery to prevent uterine inertia—which is when your labour could slow down or come to a complete halt because the muscles of the uterus are not contracting hard enough; *Caulophyllum* also helps to expel the afterbirth and soothes any discomfort afterwards.

A woman can be treated homoeopathically throughout her pregnancy even if she is going regularly to an orthodox ante-natal clinic. It is advisable to be guided by a homoeopathic doctor, since symptoms, situations and cures vary with each individual, and it is part of the essence of homoeopathy that the entire symptom picture is taken into account with each patient.

Even if you find you are seeing a different doctor each time you go to your orthodox clinic, explain that you are using homoeopathic medicine. According to my own adviser, homoeopathic cures do not conflict or interfere chemically with any other medicine or drug you might have taken.

You must tell your homoeopathic doctor if you are taking or have taken anything else because homoeopathy is concerned with the intrinsic balance of the metabolism, and strong medication could disturb this balance. For instance if you have been prescribed, and want to take, sleeping pills on an orthodox medical prescription, that drug might possibly interfere with the homoeopathic treatment— although the homoeopathic treatment would not alter the efficiency of the prescribed sleeping pills.

The Queen and the entire Royal Family are treated homoeopathically. The late Sir John Weir was the Royal Family's personal homoeopathic physician for many years, and they are now attended by Dr Margery Blackie.[1]

The correct dosage should always be checked either with a homoeopathic specialist or homoeopathic chemist. All remedies will be available through either of these sources, and come in the form of

1. Dr Blackie's book *The Patient, Not the Cure*, Macdonald and Janes, London, 1976.

white powder, or small white pills, which should be placed on the tongue in a dry mouth and allowed to dissolve. There are homoeopathic doctors available on the National Health Service in England if you can find them. Private consultants are not so difficult to trace.

HERBAL REMEDIES

'It is the Earth, like a kind mother, receives us at our birth, and sustains us when born. It is this alone, of all the elements around us, that is never found enemy to man.'

PLINY, A.D. 23–79

'The Lord hath created Medicines out of the earth; and he that is wise will not abhor them.'

ECC. XXXVIII 4.

Herbal medicine has been practised over the centuries, and our present pharmacology is based on the properties inherent in herbs. In fact, some of the tablets prescribed by doctors now are still derived from plants. Others are technically distilled or purified equivalents of the active principals in plants. However, as with natural food, there are those who prefer to take in the ingredients, particularly the vitamins, in organic form. Too much food now comes in tins and cans and frozen lumps with all the natural goodness processed out. Although a minute proportion of herbs used are toxic, at least 99 per cent are not, and have a natural balance of nutritious and healing properties.

So here are a few suggestions about natural sources of nourishment particularly important to you when expecting a baby. The things you eat keep your metabolism going, and, as we've already seen (section on diet), can cause or prevent overweight and its accompanying disorders.

Your body is a well-designed instrument, not only for carrying a child but for warding off disease. If you treat it right, the odds are it will treat you right. Although more people buy their food as packages in the supermarket now than dig them up from the ground, there are still rich sources of mineral and protein surrounding us.

Iron   One of the most important elements in the blood; iron is part of the red corpuscle essential for transporting oxygen in the blood. Lack may cause iron deficiency anaemia, paleness, run-down and weakened condition.

Find it in spinach, parsley, strawberry leaves (strawberry leaf tea is a delicious way to take it), watercress and most green vegetables. In Britain the National Health Service will provide iron and folic acid pills free during pregnancy. You will find iron in meat, but if you don't like your basic relationship with animals to be the taste of their flesh in your mouth, then try soya beans for protein and plenty of green vegetables. If you do eat meat, offal such as kidneys and liver has the most iron content.

Calcium

Needed for the formation of good bones and teeth in the baby; during pregnancy and breastfeeding women need much more than the normal amount of calcium as they must provide it for the baby as well as themselves. Traces of calcium can be found in camomile, chives, dandelion root, nettles and sorrel. Milk is much the best source, so drink a pint a day and remember to eat yoghurt and cheese.

Vitamins

Some vitamins are manufactured within plants, and herbalists believe plant vitamins or minerals are easier to digest than those of fish or animal origin.

Vitamin A

Needed for night vision and proper functioning of the cells of skin and mucous membrane.

Botanical sources: alfalfa (which should be grown for seven years to reach its full strength), dandelion, okra pods, parsley and watercress.

Carrots are an excellent source of Vitamin A, and also pumpkin.

B complex vitamins	These can be found in wholewheat breads, wheatgerm, brown rice, any whole, unprocessed cereals and particularly in dried brewer's yeast. Also present in pork, bacon, kidneys and egg yolk.
Vitamin B₁₂	Essential for the normal development of red blood cells; it is found in foods of animal origin.

Vitamin B₁₂ — Essential for the normal development of red blood cells; it is found in foods of animal origin.

Botanical sources: alfalfa if picked while sprouting, kelp and comfrey.

For a supplement you can also buy B_{12} in pill or liquid form over the counter at most chemists.

Vitamin C — Needed for healthy teeth and gums; recent research by Nobel Prize winner Linus Pauling has shown that massive doses can help ward off or get rid of the common cold and the body will rid itself of any excess; it is destroyed by heat, cooking, low temperatures and oxidation; and because it is not stored by the body, needs constant replenishment.

Botanical sources: elderberries, oregano, paprika, parsley, rose hip, watercress. Also find it in fruit like oranges, lemons and blackcurrants. *Note:* those with any allergic tendencies towards fruit acids should be careful with this vitamin as an excess could encourage thrush, cystitis and cramps.

Vitamin D — Found in fish oils such as halibut and cod liver oil. This vitamin is synthesized by ultra-violet rays on the skin. Chief source: sunlight on the skin.

Vitamin E — The major source of this vitamin is wheatgerm, but there are small amounts in many foods, particularly eggs. Some margarines contain it. Taken internally, it can help hemorrhoids.

| | It lowers the blood pressure, and should be avoided by those with any kind of rheumatic heart condition. |
| *Vitamin K* | Necessary in the physiological process of blood clotting; it helps any kind of hemorrhage and is often given after a difficult delivery. |

Botanical sources: alfalfa herb and horse chestnut leaves. Can also be found in all green vegetables, such as cabbage, peas, etc.

For the treatment of one of the great discomforts of pregnancy—hemorrhoids or piles—there are suppositories, and a horse chestnut cream ointment called Anco, made in England by A. Nelson & Company.

HERBAL TEAS

These are not only healing agents but some have a relaxing effect if you feel edgy or out of sorts emotionally. They do not have the let-down or depressing after-effects of most chemical stimulants. Herbalists would call our normal everyday Indian tea a stimulant, also coffee. That is for the purist. I list some good soothing herb teas here mainly because of their specific medicinal value in pregnancy, but also because they are delicious to drink anyway, and it's fun occasionally to try something new in the teapot!

Method: warm the pot, one ounce of herb tea per pint of boiling water. Pour on water as soon as it boils. Let the tea brew for seven minutes. Stir. Pour out after a minute. Never make teas in aluminium containers.

Alfalfa Tea

This herb is one of nature's richest sources of easily assimilated vitamins (B_{12}, E, K, and Niacin). Brew it with mint for extra flavour. To reach full strength the alfalfa crop should be allowed to grow for seven years.

Naturebirth

Camomile Tea

This is thought to be a certain remedy for nightmares and sleeplessness. Drink it before dinner with a little ginger—or afterwards with one part fennel to two parts camomile. Sweeten it with honey. Served cold it can soothe the digestion after a particularly heavy meal.

Ginger Tea

A warming tea for chills, indigestion or an upset stomach. Be careful how much you use, as ginger can be very strong. The average amount would be half a small teaspoon for one large cup, but this will vary with the strength of the ginger.

Hop Tea

Used to improve appetite and digestion, it also helps induce sleep if you have it just as you go to bed.

Labrador or Swamp Tea

This was used by the American Indians to 'soothe stomachs and aching bones'.

Linden or Lime Flower Tea

Tastes a bit like sweet jasmine and is very soothing for taut nerves after a day of aggravation.

Nettle Tea

Nettles are a rich source of iron, and nettle tea is one of the oldest recorded beverages of the English countryside, believed to have been introduced by the Romans. Mix it with ordinary tea leaves if you like a blend. It is thought by connoisseurs to be delicious. Dry nettle leaves should be rubbed through a sieve and then add one part nettle to three parts ordinary tea, and thoroughly mix. Flavour with lemon and honey. Nettles can be delicious made into soup. Cook and season as you would spinach.

Parsley Tea

Good source of vegetable iron—make as with any tea.

Raspberry Leaf Tea

This is an old European remedy especially for pregnant women which helps tone the uterus and soothes the woman. Usually indicated in the last three months of pregnancy.

Persimmon Tea and Rose Hip Tea

Rich in Vitamin C—make as with any tea.

Spearmint Tea

Good for stopping nausea and for getting rid of that yucky taste in the mouth after vomiting.

Sweet (or Slippery) Elm Tea

Especially good for upset early pregnant stomachs that cannot hold anything else down. Pour a cup of boiling water over a teaspoon of cut Slippery Elm bark. When it is cold, strain and add lemon juice and brown sugar to taste.

Make sure your diet has plenty of protein and not too much carbohydrate; with fresh fruit, vegetables and dairy products, and soya beans if you do not eat fish or meat.

Remember to cook vegetables lightly so you do not boil out the vitamins, and greens are still fibrous enough to chew on. Fibre content in food is important for roughage—regular bowel movement—and as exercise for your teeth, which need something to chew on! If you do not take care they are one of the first things to weaken during pregnancy as the baby takes so much calcium from you.

If you cannot wander over the countryside picking your own wild herbs, then substitute herbalist for hedgerows, and look for your nearest dealer in natural vitamins. In England and America you can buy bottled organic vitamins in health food stores; in America drug stores often have a shelf or two of organic drugs; London has the famous Culpeper Houses, named after the great herbalist Nicholas Culpeper, and various wholesalers such as those listed in Appendix V.

Culpeper House was in fact founded by Mrs Hilda Lewel in 1927. She also founded the Society of Herbalists, which is a lay body and registered charity and serves as an international centre for all aspects of herbalism.

It is important to stress here that, as with homoeopathy, herbal medicine can be misjudged by the inexperienced. It is always better to be under the guidance of a specialist. However, Great Britain is the only country where herbal medicine can stiill be practised under statute; and the National Institute of Medical Herbalists confers a diploma after a minimum four years training and examinations.

7

Labour Day

Labour Means Work

There is no perfect labour. What you do and what happens to you is neither right nor wrong. Better to get rid of any question of such judgements before you go into labour, or setting yourself an impossible goal may lead to needless feelings of inadequacy or let-down when the time comes. Do not imagine ecstasy and then be annoyed when you are landed with a very uncomfortable few hours at the end of which is a baby! Inevitably each one of us experiences giving birth and being born with varying degrees of emotion and physical sensation, according to individual metabolism and state of mind. There is no success and no failure—just a simple rate of progression to be aware of and some information that may prove useful.

Getting ready to have a baby is like an athlete training for the Olympics. You are preparing for a peculiarly taxing event. There are breathing exercises designed to help the uterus work freely; we extend ourselves so much in such a short space of time, so daily practice is one way to become fit and strong and accustomed to work. Labour literally means work. But it doesn't have to mean 'travail' in the old biblical sense of 'in sorrow thou shalt bring forth children'.[1] The average female body is well equipped to do this work, and hopefully bring forth children with joy.

There may be moments when you wonder how on earth your own body will stretch enough to deliver a baby. I remember, even having had a child, finding the *reality* of something as large as a baby's head

1. Genesis, 3: 16.

204

coming out of the narrow orifice between my legs, almost impossible to relate to. It becomes less scarey, when you know that nature releases various mechanisms to help your body adjust to giving birth.

For instance, it is not only you who work during labour, the baby works too. Scientists now believe it is the fetal pituitary gland which initiates the process of birth through the interaction of a series of hormones,[1] so he propels himself through the birth canal having himself stimulated your uterus to help push him out. All through pregnancy, your own glands secrete hormones which soften and extend the birth canal, and the ligaments of your pelvis accordingly relax, allowing room for slight movement between bones which are usually held securely together.[2]

Then too there is the small miracle of the baby's skull. If you touch gently the surface skin of a newborn baby's head, you will find a vulnerable little patch, through which you can see and feel his pulse beat, before the hard bones of the skull grow together. So, as he is being born, the bones are still soft enough to move, and the child's head moulds itself to the mother's available space. Sometimes this accounts for temporarily odd-shaped heads, but they expand and round out and generally right themselves amazingly quickly considering the pressure—usually within a few days.

The pattern of labour can be divided very roughly into three parts, according to doctors. First the dilation and thinning of the cervix until the cervix is fully opened; second the crowning and delivery of the baby; third the delivery of the placenta, the afterbirth. This is tremendously simplified for the observer. A woman in labour should know the more detailed progression of events.

When labour starts the baby is usually facing his mother's right side with his arms and legs flexed. His head has already dropped into the pelvis far enough for there to be a difference in the woman's pregnant silhouette. Now there is a visible space between the football that is the belly and the breasts. His head is what the medical profession call 'engaged'—in other words, lying low in the pelvic

1. G. S. Dawes, Director of the Nuffield Institute of Medical Research, Oxford University, writing on 'The Hazards of Birth in Human Reproduction' in the *Science Journal*, London, 1971, p. 135.
2. *Birth of a Baby*, Marshall Cavendish Learning System: *Man and Medicine*, 1969, p. 31.

basin and just about ready to go. But the cervix is still thick and the membranes intact.

In some labours, the membranes rupture early and this breaking of the waters starts the descent of the baby's head into the birth canal, and, more important, stimulates contractions. Sometimes, if the bag of waters seems to be forming a barrier for the descent of the child's head, the membrane will be ruptured by the doctor.

The first thing which happens is that the cervix begins to stretch and thin with very mild early labour contractions. For this you can use the first level 'A' breathing.[1] Then the cervix actually begins to dilate or open, becoming thinner as it pulls back over the baby's head. For this you can use the next breathing levels, 'A' through 'B' to 'C'. Then contractions become longer and more intense as the cervix becomes more dilated. Now you may want to use level 'D' breathing as well. The next stage is tricky. Those teaching psychoprophylaxis, or natural birth, call it 'transition', although it is not a recognized medical term, it is a good word to describe the period of time—anything from a few minutes to about two hours—during which the uterus is preparing to expel the baby, but the baby's head is not yet 'crowning' (becoming visible), so you must not push.

There is a special type of breathing for transition which helps to prevent you pushing, even though you feel you want to. When you get the go-ahead to push, the baby's head will usually be the first thing to appear, this is called 'crowning', and delivery should follow with the next few contractions. The final step is the expulsion of the placenta.

TRANSITION

That stage of labour described as 'transition' needs a special explanation. It is one of the most difficult parts of labour, both physically and emotionally. You have probably been dealing with contractions for quite a while now, and really want to *do* something about getting that baby out of you and into the air where he wants to be. But you cannot push. You have to hold back. Transition means the passage from one state or set of circumstances to another. Therein lies the key. You are about to move from the state of labour to the state of delivery. Your cervix is almost completely dilated and

1. See Appendix I for breathing techniques.

the baby's head right down in the birth canal, just about to move into the open, yet not quite ready. Although you may want to push, you are told you must not. The head is not quite far enough down the birth canal and the cervix has not drawn back fully over the head. Pushing now could damage your cervix and the baby. It feels very peculiar and for this reason you can use a particular pattern of breathing to help divert the urge to push until you are fully dilated.

Transition is an emotional blockbuster. Freak out. You feel awful. Everybody does. It is actually a signal that things are about to move on but while you are going through it, you'll need to be reminded of what is happening very lovingly, because you may be feeling bitchy, angry, despairing and tearful and, most of all, very very tired. Remember this flood of emotion is a perfectly normal part of the pattern.

If you have held off drugs until this point, try to keep it together for a bit longer. Transition does not last. And the stage it moves into is the moment of birth. So try to look forward instead of back, even though you feel as if you simply can't go on, you want to pack your bags and walk out of the door never to return. But as long as your mediating man is there to understand what's happening, you should be able to get through it without tearing up the delivery room, punching the nurses or breaking up your marriage. Whoever is helping you must remember that if you yell for dope now, wanting anything that's going to numb the waves of feeling washing over you, when anyone touching you is a monster and if one more of these damned contractions hits you you'll just give up and not have the baby at all—the situation is not as desperate as you make it sound and he can nudge you gently through the crisis with the reminder that it is nearly over. The baby is nearly there.

Unfortunately, it has been my experience, and that of too many of my friends, that some nurses are indifferent, or unable to relate to a woman's emotions in labour, and very often will not believe a woman when she says her baby is coming. Do not allow anyone to override your own instincts. We all have a tendency to believe the people in uniform are the people who know, although experience shows it isn't always the case. Many nurses have no personal experience of giving birth to go by, and perhaps their medical training puts little emphasis on the importance of sensitivity. For whatever reason, they are often reluctant to listen to a woman stating her own case during labour. Prepared women usually deal with contractions quite calmly. They feel in control of the situation. This again is strange to medical staff who are accustomed to soothing maternal hysteria with drugs. Should you question the system or refuse the usual medication, you become 'difficult'. A nuisance. A threat to the established order.

One maternity hospital, run by nuns, at which I attended a birth, estimated they had forty sedated or anaesthetized births to one 'natural' labour and delivery. Consequently they were amazed, and in some peculiar way, affronted, when the woman I was with insisted on managing her own labour rather than use tranquillizing drugs.

When my youngest son was born I started to have the overwhelming desire to push which usually signals the baby's imminent arrival. The urge came much sooner than any of us had expected—I had been in the delivery room for only two hours. I told the doctor I wanted to bear down. He said, 'Oh no, not yet.' Then felt to see how dilated the cervix was—reluctant even to examine me so soon. Looked surprised, nodded, said, 'You can push with the next contraction', removed his gloves and walked out of the room saying 'You'll have the baby in about half an hour'. He had obviously found the cervix fully dilated, but didn't believe I was ready to deliver.

As the next contraction swept over me I held in my breath ready to push, and absolutely knew the baby was about to come out. I shouted out for the doctor to come back, but he had left the room. The nurse ran for the bell to summon him, leaving no one between my legs to help deliver the baby's head. John was supporting my knees. He let go and leapt to the end of the bed as his son's head shot out wetly into his waiting hands!

I think the most important thing to remember about transition, especially with first babies—when you have already had one child, your muscles are not so tight and you know more about what to do—is that you need to breathe in a way that *stops* you from doing exactly what you feel like doing. When there's a good reason for you not to push, you have to be able to re-route the urge. It is confusing because you can feel two things going on. The neck of the uterus is still opening with the contractions, as it has throughout labour, but you can also feel it flexing and preparing for the next stage—the expulsion of the baby. Now his face is turned towards your back, in a normal delivery, and he is about to pop out. You have to redirect your breathing from the need to push out, into another channel where it can actually prevent you from pushing out. The breathing you can learn to help do this is called: 'Blow, one two, one two'.[1]

Transition can also be handled lying on your side. Some midwives prefer to deliver this way, especially in Europe, so it is important to check with your doctor or hospital beforehand and find out if you are likely to be ordered into this position. If so, and you do not feel uncomfortable, take the pillows away from your head and move onto your side for transition, so that when the baby's head crowns you are ready.

Lie in a crescent shape with one pillow under your head and one under your shoulder. Put the arm touching the bed forward, in front of your body, and the opposite upper leg forward with a pillow for support so that your thigh is at right angles to the rest of your body—then put the upper arm along the upper thigh. Go up through the levels of breathing till you get to level 'D'. When you get the pushing urge, slide that hand along your thigh till it is past the knee so that your chest is in the same slump as in the sitting position when you expel the air. Bring the hand back up the thigh, count 'one two, one two', and then slump again.

You can lie on your side on the floor for the 'blow, one two, one two' exercise, and experiment with positions for arms and legs. It is a good idea if the conductor of a preparation group sees first that everyone is comfortable with pillows supporting heads and shoulders, one under the belly for extra comfort or one under the upper leg which is thrown forward. Then when you say 'blow', the top arm should go forward in front of the body with the exhaled breath, then, counting 'one two, one two' the arm pulls back again to rest along the side.

Personally the thought of lying on my side, or indeed lying down at all during labour was anathema. I wanted to be propped up enough to see what was going on, stay awake and stay on top of contractions with my breathing. The very thought of sinking down made me feel suffocated. I thought I would lose touch with myself.

In practice I found it sent me immediately to sleep. I think I found it too awkward to even want to handle. But some people find

1. See Appendix I for transition breathing exercises.

it more comfortable than sitting up, especially if they are feeling contractions in their back or thighs.

If you are already on your side for a side delivery, all you have to do when the baby starts coming is pick up at the knee the leg that is thrown forward, supporting it with the crook of the arm that is on the floor, and you have a perfect arch for your baby to pass through.

'CROWNING' OF THE BABY'S HEAD AND DELIVERY

As the baby is being pushed down through the birth canal by the combined force of the uterine contractions and your voluntary bearing-down efforts, the top of his head can be seen at the opening of the vagina. His head is 'crowning'.

If his father stands at the end of the bed, he'll see the top of a tiny head trying to come out. The woman, if she is fully conscious, will be pushing, using all her force, determination and energy to direct her abdominal muscles in the final effort of labour. The child's face is usually turned completely towards his mother's back. The mother's perineum is stretched and, with the vulva, bulges like a crown over the baby's emerging brow and head. The muscles of the abdominal wall are still contracting, and the perineum becomes extremely thin. The mother should not push too hard at this stage in case she should tear. A tear could be superficial and harmless, or it could run jaggedly from vagina to rectum, and it is the risk of this which would be a viable reason for performing an episiotomy. The top of the baby's head then moves right out of the vagina and the mother's perineum will shrink back to its more normal appearance. The baby's body continues to turn. The contracting wall of the uterus fits like a cap over his buttocks, the head turns upwards and the pelvic floor slips back over his face. You can see him!

Now the doctor rotates the shoulders while the baby's body is still inside, gently supporting the head all the time. As contractions continue and you push out the rest of his body, the doctor guides the head away. The baby may start breathing now, or even cry out, though this may not happen until his body has completely emerged.

A newborn baby's head is not the round fluffy little powder puff you might fondly imagine. It can look quite odd, to say the least, and if forceps or a suction cap have been used to pull him out, the head may look particularly pointed or swollen or bruised in some way.

That soon subsides, so do not let it worry you. But his skull will be damp and babies' heads come in a variety of colours, from mauve to grey to blue. The vernix cream, which is probably all over his body too, will make any hair he has look white and sticky.

There is nearly always a short interval of perhaps a minute between the birth of the baby's head and the shoulders. This helps you, because you get a few moments' rest before that last push which produces your whole infant, and gives your child a precious period of adjustment, so that he may get a little used to the sensations of the world outside your womb. Sometimes the midwife will take this chance to wipe the mucus from his mouth and nose before he takes his first breath. Sometimes the mucus has to be sucked out with a tube. The first 'prepared' baby of mine, Orion, had the cord round his neck three times as he came out and the doctor stepped in and slipped it from around his neck before any damage could be done. It happened so quickly I scarcely had time to register the danger. The third child, Liam (second 'prepared' birth), was born very easily and breathed while his body was still inside me. I watched his eyes open in alert awareness well before his whole body slipped out of mine, then held him in my arms with the vernix still covering him, and the cord still joining us.

A woman's relaxed and natural participation during delivery is twofold. First she is helping things along by maintaining a good supply of oxygen for uterus and baby through breathing correctly, and secondly she is reinforcing the natural expulsion of the baby from the uterus by being aware enough to utilize contractions for pushing. Without the slowing down effect of sedatives, and with the active help of the woman pushing for herself, in a normal labour the uterus is unlikely to take any longer to do its job than is healthy for mother or child.

Contractions at this point of delivery are much shorter and more frequent than in the earlier parts of labour. It is much more comfortable for a woman if she can be propped up with pillows rather than lying flat on her back. This way she is supported at her spine, and can see what is going on. In Appendix I you will see the exact level of breathing needed to help delivery. At the same time as you breathe through contractions, lift up both legs at the knee so your feet are raised to help delivery. Put your arms along the sides of the bed, then, keeping the elbows flat to take the weight of the legs, tuck your hands under your knees and lift. Knowing how to do this yourself, or being able to get your birth assistant to help you, means there is really no excuse for putting you into stirrups for delivery. Stirrups are uncomfortable, awkward and necessitate lying flat on your back with your legs waving in the air. By holding up your legs yourself, you achieve the same result, which is to make it easy for the baby to come out, in the most natural and comfortable way (see illustration in Appendix I, page 271).

Don't let anyone persuade you to press the soles of your feet against them. Sometimes nurses take your feet in their hands and urge you to press. This is quite wrong. If you have had someone hold the base of your feet you'll realize how ticklish it can be, and the physical reaction to someone tickling your soles is to draw back and tense up. Since you are trying to do the opposite when you are delivering a baby—no nurses at the bottom of your feet!

The baby is usually born covered in the vernix cream. Try to remember to ask the doctor or the midwife to leave it on. It nourishes and lubricates and protects his skin. Usually babies are taken away and scrubbed up before being given back to the mother. Try just wiping mouth, nose and eyes with a little warm olive oil, leaving the vernix on the skin for as long as possible.

The baby will change colour again when he takes over his own breathing. Most babies are born a purple or bluish colour. When they stop using the umbilical cord as their life source, and breathe for themselves instead, they gradually become pink. For the first time, oxygenated blood from the baby's own lungs is racing around his body. This is when he most needs physical contact with his mother, before the gap between the two widens so far that it cannot be bridged. Ask the midwife to hand you your baby while he is still attached to you by the umbilical cord and then you won't break contact in those first vital moments of his life. If you already have children, you know that to touch a child is to comfort. How much more powerful that touch must be at birth, to assure this new being that, although physically separated from your flesh, he is not as lost as he might feel, experiencing his own weight for the first time, unsupported in this new element, air, after the familiar liquid warmth of your womb home. You too can assuage that curious sense of loss as the child leaves your body, by touching him gently and holding him close.

After the birth of the baby, the uterus continues to contract, the walls become thicker and the cavity gets smaller. Since the placenta and the amniotic membrane cannot contract, and the inner surface of the uterus to which they are attached is getting smaller, they are separated and expelled in what doctors call the delivery of the afterbirth. This usually takes place within an hour, often much less, of the baby's delivery. Some people are lucky and the placenta comes shooting out without any trouble minutes after the baby. Others aren't so lucky and it can sometimes take longer than an hour. The midwife may press on your stomach to stimulate the contractions and you will have to use your breathing exercises again. If it takes longer than an hour, the doctor will intervene himself and it may mean having a short general anaesthetic. Over an hour is an unusually long time and means the placenta may still be attached in part to the lining of the womb, or may have broken loose, but be tightly gripped by the contractions of the womb. If there is a delay you will normally be given an injection of oxytocin, the hormone used for inducing labour artificially, which is released in your own body naturally when you go into spontaneous labour. Its action is to stimulate the uterus into contracting. With this and some very gentle pulling on the cord the afterbirth should come away satisfactorily. It is only in rare cases that a woman would have to be anaesthetized.

The uterus is much smaller, once it has delivered the child. While delivering the afterbirth it becomes hard and moves up into the top part of the abdomen again, above the navel. Oxytocin or ergometrine or syntocinon, a mixture of both now commonly used, helps hold the uterus firmly contracted to prevent excess bleeding. Straight away after labour, the uterus starts to return to its normal size and shape. By somewhere between the fourteenth and the twenty-first day after delivery, the lining has healed completely and by six weeks the uterus is back to almost its original size.

POSSIBLE DELIVERY COMPLICATIONS

Posterior-position Baby

When they tell you your baby is in a posterior position, don't worry too much; this is not very unusual, but on the other hand, it is not the position in which most babies start labour. His head is down, but instead of the crown of his head to the fore, ready to take the full brunt of pushing through the birth canal, the back of his head is towards your back and he is facing the front of your body. It can mean a somewhat longer first stage of labour, possibly with back ache, as his head rotates to come round into the usual position for delivery. Sometimes the doctor will try to help this manually and sometimes the child is actually born face first.

Breech-position Baby

This means he is the wrong way round and isn't ready to come out head first in the usual way. The baby is either 'flexed' which means he's curled up into a ball, or 'extended' with the legs stretched up straight, feet above shoulders. This makes it more difficult for him to negotiate the curve of the birth canal, and the obstetrician usually unhooks the legs just before the actual birth. Often the doctor will be able to turn the baby the right way round in the weeks before delivery. If not, you will probably be encouraged to give birth to your child's body first, and then your doctor may lift the baby's legs up over your belly to help out the head as quickly as possible. Now you know the physiology, and have a general outline for the progression of labour, you need to know what to look for when your own labour is about to begin.

First Signs of Labour

The first signs of labour are light contractions. Of course, you say. But you might be having mild contractions on and off during the last weeks of pregnancy, so it may be difficult to recognize the real thing. When labour is starting, the twinges come regularly and feel like extreme period pains, a sort of ache around the base of your spine or lower abdomen, as though fingers were tugging insistently at the innermost strings of your being.

Before you have entered labour proper, the faint contractions you detect are just the uterus flexing itself from time to time, getting ready for labour. You can use the first level of breathing when that happens, but the sensation won't last long or feel very strong. When labour contractions begin, you'll know by their regularity and be able to see the muscles harden just beneath the skin of your stomach. It looks like a fist clenching.

Most people think you have to time the period between contractions. In fact it is how long the contraction lasts that is important in telling you how far along you are. And then later, the intensity strengthens as you progress. Light contractions at the beginning of labour last about thirty seconds, the stronger ones a little longer. Even the mild contractions seem to take quite a long time. Practising the breathing with a watch before you go into labour gives you an idea of how much energy you will use (see Appendix I for breathing pattern).

People tend to laugh off early contractions because they've been waiting for them for such a long time. I remember weeks too early mistaking cramps for indigestion and the baby's kick for contractions. You build up and build up in anticipation so that when the real ones start it is hard to believe they are happening.

Another signal is that you get a huge rush of energy suddenly. Perhaps you are constantly energetic, but pregnancy usually afflicts you with a certain lassitude in its weighty waiting time. The rush can bring you wide awake and have you whizzing around cleaning cupboards or sorting bookshelves, even if it is the middle of the night.

I can remember each time tearing around like a speed freak and having to be physically restrained, so that I was rested enough to deal with the remainder of labour. I looked in the mirror once and was astonished to see I looked orange. It must have been extra blood racing to the surface of my skin, but it was quite amazing to see myself turn the colour of a Mediterranean sunset.

The more you can rest at the beginning of labour, the better for you. If it is at night, which happens often, and you can get back to sleep, fine. If you can't, don't take a pill, that will just make you dopey and drowsy so later, when you want to be wide awake to cope with strong contractions, you won't be. Just get your feet up, relax, read, play board games, watch television, do whatever you find the most restful, soothing and comfortable. Conserving energy is vital now.

Your bladder is getting a great deal of pressure from the baby so you'll want to pee frequently. You may also get diarrhea. Nervous excitement has the same effect. It's quite lucky if you do get diarrhea —it may avoid having waste forcibly washed out of you by an enema when you get to the hospital. (One of the more unpleasant memories of childbirth in an English hospital.)

The next thing to look for when you are still at home is a 'show'. This is when the plug of mucus that has formed at the mouth of the womb to protect the baby from infection, comes away to make room for the baby's head starting its journey down the birth canal. The plug is just like a small lump of clear jelly, slightly streaked with red blood. Note the time you see it, so you can tell the hospital or doctor.

Then the membranes may either break or leak. A leak is just like a thimbleful of warm clear liquid pouring out of your vagina—and is another signal that labour is getting under way. Very often the membranes do not rupture until you are well advanced in labour and then the baby's head, pressing down hard on the bag of waters, eventually breaks it. In some women this happens early and feels like a flood of lukewarm water streaming between your legs. It is not comparable to peeing because there is absolutely no control over it, and in this case there will be about two cupfuls, rather than the thimbleful that comes with a 'leak'. If you have a thick-skinned sac it may have to be broken by the doctor later. But don't think because you haven't felt any kind of leak it means you aren't in labour. The most reliable way of telling is by the length and strength of contractions.

Start using level 'A' breathing[1] as soon as you feel them, then you can judge calmly when you need to go up another level to 'B'. Remember to let go and flow into the sensation if contractions seem to hurt. Remember to relax, relax, relax—write it on the back of your hand or the wall or behind your old man's ear where only you can see such private messages—then if you let go instead of tightening up, muscle tension won't be opposing the dilation of the cervix. You'll be surprised at how much difference simply knowing that you have become tense makes to your ability to let go.

One of the best things you can do before your waters break is have a bath. It is utterly relaxing, lots of bubbles and good smells pamper you, and the warmth not only acts as a stimulant to contractions, but may, by increasing the circulation of blood to the abdomen, make the transition from weak to stronger contractions easier. Don't lock the door while you have a bath, and don't when you go to the lavatory. It's unlikely that you'll desperately need help, but if you should, then it must be easy for someone to get to you. It is also a

1. Appendix I.

216

bad idea to have a bath if you are alone in the house. Some labours can be amazingly quick. Especially if it is a third or fourth baby when neither muscle nor psychic tension is so pronounced. You may step into the tub breathing lightly in level 'A' and suddenly be overtaken by stronger contractions and need a helping hand out of the water. It is just a common-sense precaution that for a woman in labour help should be accessible at all times.

If you feel hungry, have a light meal perhaps, but try to stick to nourishing fluids, preferably something with honey in it. You will need as much energy as you can muster in the next few hours. Also remember that hospitals do not usually have anywhere for visitors to eat, so if you are going into hospital, and your man is going too, he should have something to eat at this stage. Whatever you eat should be easy to digest. Digestion is reduced to a minimum during labour. You need to stock up on energy reserves like an engine needs stoking, but it is important not to overdo it, or rather to choose sensibly the fuel you use. A solid starchy meal could land you in trouble, should you need to have an anaesthetic. Being anaesthetized on top of food could cause vomiting and then choking, which could possibly be fatal. That is why they always tell you not to eat before going to the dentist, or before you have an operation.

The available sugar in your bloodstream gets used up very quickly by the strenuous physical effort of labour. This is why it is a good thing to take honey in some form or another, either by the spoonful, or stirred into a soothing tea. It can be absorbed in large quantities without upsetting the digestive system, and has the highest concentrated natural sugar content. We took a pot of delicious orange blossom honey into hospital with us, and I would just eat a spoonful of it in between contractions. Glucose tablets, too, are easily absorbed into the bloodstream, and a good energy boost. I nibbled handfuls of them in the early part of labour to no ill effect. So did John. I'd advise getting in a store of packets so they're there if you want them.

In the late stages of labour, indigestion or wind can make things uncomfortable. Some people burp, some get hiccups, some don't realize they are doing it, some feel so undignified that it ties them in knots while it's happening. Don't let it. Wind is quite normal. It has to escape and when you are in labour there's less room for it than at any other time. Again, if you keep your solid food intake down, it is less likely to happen; fruit juices, vegetable juices, broth, milk or tea with lots of honey is the best answer.

Be prepared for cold extremities. Fingers and nose can get chilly, but particularly feet. Socks take care of cold toes, so make sure you look out a warm woolly pair before labour is due, so you can put them on once contractions begin. You'd be surprised at what a difference it makes to relaxation to keep your feet warm. Sometimes you can get chills all over. If you do get the shakes, cover up as warm as you can—I remember asking for a hot water bottle, but it is apparently against hospital policy to give people hot water bottles, in case they burst and the hospital gets sued for malpractice or something. You could try taking your own hot water bottle with you; of course if you are at home you don't have anything to worry about. Something warm at the base of your spine would be enormously comforting during normal contractions too. Some people suggest putting an ice-pack there if you are getting contractions in your back rather than belly—but I must say I just wanted to keep warm. An important thing to remember about shaking during contractions is that, as with the administration of an enema and shaving the pubic hairs, if you move into the sensation instead of bracing against it, you will find that after a bit the shivers go right through you and away again like a passing storm. If you clench your teeth and fists and try to stop it that way, you will make things much worse.

If you find a contraction coming over you while you are in the bath or on the lavatory or having a drink or packing your things or whatever it is you are doing when labour begins—then just drop everything and deal with the contraction with level 'A' (the first level) breathing. This level is usually enough until contractions become longer and more intense. When it gets to the stage when you are using level 'B', or you have had a 'show' and either a leak or rupture of the membranes, then it is time to telephone the midwife, if you are at home, and the hospital or doctor if you are due to go into hospital.

If you have to ring the hospital, ask to be put through to the Maternity Ward, or Labour Ward Sister. She'll ask you how long your contractions are, when they started, how much time there is between them and if or when you had a 'show'. That way she will be able to tell when to instruct you to come into hospital.

An ambulance usually takes about ten minutes to get to you in a large city like London. But it is wise to check that beforehand. If you are being driven there by car, do a dry run before you go into labour to get an idea of how long it takes. It is usually more comfortable for people to travel facing the engine, so if you go by ambulance, ask the driver to take you in feet first so you don't have your back to the engine.

It is pretty exciting by this time. No more rehearsals, this is it, the big day. You feel nervous and excited at the same time. It's like entering a huge competition you're not even sure you want to be in. If you are at all like me, you'll have a dry mouth, prickles up your spine and a churning stomach. However prepared you are, the thrill is bound to get to you—so be ready for that too! It's so good to be able to hold a friendly hand. If your man is not there, try to make sure someone is. Someone you like and trust who knows about your training and can help you keep to your breathing.

If you are having your baby at home, one of the key advantages is that the atmosphere is relaxing. When contractions start you can just fall into your own bed, having bathed in your own bath and eaten at your own table. If you are having to organize everything to move from your home into hospital, then there are bound to be things to do and situations to cope with, even if it is something like sitting in a cramped car in a traffic jam trying to get to the hospital. So be ready to use your breathing under any circumstances, and be unembarrassed to opt out of whatever is happening around you.

Now, about those things to take into hospital with you. The hospital will give you a list of essentials, but there are also a few neat innovations which I discovered really come in handy. So here is a combination of the two, so that you can set them aside well before you think you might go into labour. It is wisest to avoid last-minute panics.

For you:

You will need an old, or dispensable nightdress to wear in labour; but have one that opens at the neck so that you can put the baby to the breast without trouble as soon as you want. Then pretty bedclothes to wear after the baby is born.

suggestions: three pretty nightdresses, which undo at the neck

two bedjackets

one dressing-gown or house robe

one pair of slippers

three nursing bras which undo in the front and can be adjusted at the back to accommodate your expanding milk-filled breasts—and they will get much bigger than in pregnancy

a supply of disposable paper pants, sanitary towels, hairbrush, comb, face flannel, toothbrush, toothpaste, Kleenex, cotton wool, nail brush, soap, talcum powder, scent, hairpins, flowers, candles, incense, shawls . . . whatever you think might make the stay in hospital more home-like.

Extras for labour:

woollen socks—comfortable, large and warm, to keep your feet from freezing when the main circulation of blood is going to the stomach

two small natural sponges—get them at the cosmetic counter of a good pharmacy (and make sure they don't give you the imitation kind which don't do the trick at all and taste horrible)—these are for wetting your lips during labour when the breathing makes them very dry, but you are usually not allowed water to drink— a sponge softens your mouth, keeps it moist, and gives you something to suck on during the last stages when it is a comfort to have something to do with your mouth while the uterus and vagina are under such pressure

Evian water in an aerosol can—this is a refresher during labour—like a cool sea mist a squirt from this mineral water onto your face will brace you, wake you, freshen you if you are getting sweaty with all the hard work. Buy it at the cosmetic counter of large stores or at a good pharmacy; it is made in France as a face treatment, and can be used for that after the baby is born—

much better than washing your face, and it keeps you cool in hot weather

soft face flannel—put this in iced water (ask the nurses for a bowl of ice) for wiping your forehead and anything else that gets sticky

lip gloss, cream or Vaseline—this helps keep your lips moist and your mouth supple

Freezella—this is a plastic container for ice cubes and some people use it as a sort of cold back pack during contractions if they have a back-ache

elastic band—to tie back long or thick hair if it starts falling over your face and making you hot

pot of honey—glucose tablets—for extra energy in the first stage of labour

For the baby:

If your child is born in hospital, they usually like to keep the baby in hospital clothes until you leave, but you must take warm clothes with you for when you both come out. Do not forget that he has only ever been inside you, insulated by your body heat, and inside hospital, which is usually pretty warm. When the baby meets the outside air for the first time it is an extreme temperature change. Make sure you've got:

two vests

nappies (either towelling or the good disposable ones)

socks or little boots

dress or button-through jump suit (called 'Babygro' in England); on the whole it is wisest to avoid synthetic materials for the baby's first weeks as they may increase the heat in hot weather, and fail to keep him warm if it is cold

shawl or jacket (depending on the time of year and climate)

*   *   *

In the case of a home delivery, it is advisable that you arrange to have someone with you twenty-four hours a day to help for the first two weeks after having the baby. You will need that time to rest and get to know your child, and you shouldn't be left alone. Whoever is helping you over this period should be able to cook, shop, change and wash nappies, keep the house warm, bath the baby and make the beds. The less a new mother has to do and worry about, the more time she has to devote to her own and the baby's health, and their relationship to one another.

Try organizing your friends and relatives before the event, to help with jobs around the house. There is a tendency for people to enjoy dropping in to take part in the celebration, but not to stay and help clear up. If you can find no one to help on a regular basis the local health authority, at least in England, will generally send you a Home Help. This doesn't cost much, about the same as for a daily cleaner in your area—and sometimes the fees can be adjusted to income in special cases. A *Which?* survey (June 1971) on maternity care in England showed 90 per cent of home-birth mothers satisfied with the care they received, as opposed to 74 per cent satisfied with care received in hospital. Most women find that midwives encourage use of natural childbirth methods and like to have the father of the child present, during birth, and helping take care of mother and child afterwards.

In order to assuage any personal doubts or anxieties, everyone contemplating a home delivery should ascertain from the attending doctor exactly how much help, medical back-up is available—and where from, and should also check with the nearest maternity hospital or clinic that there is a bed available at the due time if necessary, and that the hospital is easily accessible in emergency.

All medical necessities, along with a list for the mother's personal provisions, will be provided by the midwife approximately a month before delivery is expected. Doctor and midwife will visit the home to make sure conditions are hygienic and suitable. The health visitor for the area will visit after the birth. Requirements from parents are simple: space, cleanliness and running water. The midwife may be equipped with gas and air, Pethidine, episiotomy scissors and even an oxygen tent.

Here is a list of necessities for which to prepare for a home delivery. But remember your most valuable asset is common sense.

The midwife will leave a 'box' with the mother approximately four weeks before the baby is due. This includes sanitary towels, cotton wool, one waterproof sheet, one delivery sheet, umbilical cord ligatures and dressings.

The mother provides:

> two large basins (one for the mother, one for the midwife)
> soap in a dish (for the midwife)
> two clean jam jars (one for nailbrush, one for thermometer)
> one hand towel (for midwife)
> one bucket for soiled dressings
> two one-pint jugs (one for hot water, one for cold water)
> one large sheet of clean brown paper
> one plastic sheet (approximately 2 × 1 yards)
> one large bottle of Savlon or Dettol (as a disinfectant)
> one nail brush
> one bedpan or chamber pot—or even a large plastic bucket

For herself, in labour and afterwards, I would suggest the mother equips herself with the items suggested for hospital delivery.

For the baby:

> soft bath towel to wrap the baby in after he is born
> baby bath or large wash-hand basin
> two face cloths
> two soft bath towels
> baby soap (or bath bubbles)
> baby powder
> cotton wool
> Vaseline
> surgical spirit (for cleaning cord)
> four cot sheets
> four cot blankets
> shawls
> four vests
> four nightdresses and/or Babygro (the button-through jump suits)
> at least two dozen towelling or disposable nappies
> one plastic bucket for dumping the dirties before washing

one packet of disinfectant soap powder for soiled
    nappies, clothes and bed clothes
three pairs of plastic pants (to wear over nappies)
three cardigans
bootees, bonnets and mittens (for winter babies)
one carry-cot, or cot with safety mattress
one plastic-backed towelling apron to wear while
    bathing baby
baby hair brush and comb
cotton wool swabs
nappy pins

If she will be bottle-feeding:

four (eight-ounce) bottles
six teats
plastic spoon and knife
one bucket with lid, or a Milton tank
one large bottle of Milton sterilizing fluid, or sterilizing
    tablets
measuring jug
several tins of powdered milk
bottle brush and salt (for cleaning teats)

Note: It is advisable to have these things, even if you are breast-feeding; then, if you have trouble feeding, contract an infection or have any doubts as to whether the baby is getting enough milk, especially as he gets older, you could give him a supplementary bottle and see how he takes it. If you find this relieves his hunger and stops him crying, you could give a little extra bottled milk when you feel yourself to have less—usually late in the day once you are up and about. Do look for the brands which most closely simulate human milk.

Labour of Love

*'If I want something I stretch out . . . if I'm afraid, I pull in. I go
out in love, I withdraw in anxiety . . .'*

WILHELM REICH

If you do have to go into hospital, there will most probably be a fairly rigid regime to which you will be subjected. Knowing beforehand how to deal with each situation will help make it more bearable, even if you find it impossible to change the system.

For a start, you don't have to get up in your Sunday best. They won't mind much about how you look, and will probably whip off your own clothes and put you into a regulation hospital gown anyway. But do take pillows and blankets with you if you are going to hospital by car; and don't let go of the pillows, once you get to the hospital. The staff may regard extra cushioning with impatient disapproval. Produce anything unusual, and you must be prepared to fight for your right to have it. Don't let your essential extra pillows bite the dust with your can of Evian water and pot of honey. You, after all, are the one who is having a baby. Do not let yourself be brought down by resistance to your way of having a child. Men are vital at this point. Few nurses can resist a man in labour!

When you arrive, you will be directed to the admissions room to register. Whoever is with you may be asked to give an account of himself or herself, describe the relationship to you, and, if not your legally recognized spouse, may be asked to leave. Do be firm. If there is resistance to having a helper with you, point out that with someone to assist you, there is less pressure on the nursing staff.

Next, you are likely to be whisked away, put on a bed, heaving stomach bared, and extensively examined by the midwife. She will take your temperature and blood pressure to check that all is as it should be, and listen to the baby's heart through a metal stethoscope.

Then comes the shaving of pubic hair. You may ask them to leave these hairs, but, in Britain at least, they will almost certainly insist on stubbling you along the lips of your vagina. If you get a contraction while it is happening, relax completely and move towards her hand rather than withdrawing. This will help you deal with it and help her get on with it as quickly as possible.

Exactly the same mental-cum-physical technique applies during the internal examination to see how dilated the cervix has become, and also for the administering of the enema. By moving towards and accepting what is happening, it becomes less of an intrusion.

Your hospital might use suppositories, little laxative bum rockets which have the same effect as an enema but with less discomfort. Avoid the dilemma of the bladder by making yourself get up to pee at least every hour. Get your man to remind you, if he's there. If you have to stay in bed for any reason, ask for a bedpan. Otherwise truck

225

along to the lavatory regularly. Often you do not actually feel the sensation of a full bladder when you are in labour, which is why it is a good thing to be reminded by someone else. The baby's head is pressing so hard on everything that you don't notice your bladder filling up. But a full bladder can get very painful during contractions, because to some extent it is counteracting the opening movement of the cervix.

If you find you actually can't pee, don't panic. Just sit and wait. If you are at home, you are less likely to be tense anyway, but breathing will help, as will remembering to let go the internal muscles when you breathe out. Try sitting on the lavatory with your feet on the floor and breathe through the next contraction. When it's gone, do the pelvic floor elevator exercise,[1] consciously pull in and let go the internal muscles circling the vagina.

Your geographical location in the hospital will depend at which stage of labour you are when you come in. If you are in a private room, or the first-stage labour ward, make sure you have everything needed to keep you awake. That is the only way you'll be able to stay on top of what is happening and in touch with yourself.

If it is night time, put the lights on and say 'thank you, no' nicely to the nurse who comes in with the doctor's knock-out pills. Almost any sedation now might confuse you. If you are finding labour worse than you thought, and feel you need something, ask for half the normal dose of Pethidine (50 mg). It will take the edge off sensation, but won't do you in. As this is a mood-continuing drug, it's a very good idea to have it while you feel on top of things rather than waiting till there's a hint of desperation, in which case it is the desperate mood that will continue.

Whether at home or in hospital, at this stage your man could read to you, tell you funny stories, sing lullabies, remind you of your breathing pattern, play card games, put iced water beside the bed in which to dip the flannel and sponges to cool you down and freshen you up, smooth Vaseline or cream into your lips to soften your mouth, periodically check the muscles of your face—particularly mouth, jaw and forehead—to make sure they are relaxed, powder your stomach and gently administer 'effleurage' during strong contractions.

I think it is better to save the Evian water spray for as long as

1. For pelvic floor exercise see Appendix I, p. 249.

possible, then it comes as a beautiful surprise in the steam of labouring limbs, like rain in the desert. If he thinks you are getting too sleepy or too sticky—leave the spraying to his judgement. He may want to give himself a quick shower. Assisting at labour is not cool work.

When you find your spot on the wall as an eye focus, that creeping crack in the plaster, the knob at the end of the bed, that shaft of sun on the top of a tree, the Picasso print, the slowly moving hands of a clock—tell him what it is and where it is so that if he sees your lids fluttering down, head falling or twisting from side to side away from reality and contact with the external world—he can bring you back, nudge you gently through the breathing, refocus the attention of your runaway eyes.

When you reach transition and become impossible for anyone else to deal with, he'll know it is transition, know that it is normal for you to feel like packing your bags and walking out. He can remind you that you can't—that you are going to have the baby whether you like it or not—without incurring the wrath of the gods.

If you are told you can't push, then your man, or helper, can remind you about 'blow, one two, one two'. And get you sitting up higher to deal with it. This is where the extra pillows come in very handy. They prop you up firmly. When you are directed to use the next contraction to start to push your child out of you, the wild excitement of the moment might make you forget to hold your breath, and block it with your chin on your chest. So your man just reaches for your chin and tucks it into your chest, counting with you to ten, directing your strength into using the right muscles, because he's there with you, pushing and breathing and feeling and waiting, waiting for the great moment.

He can help you hold up your feet for delivery so that if you are in hospital you aren't shoved into the hideous discomfort of stirrups. Even if you are alone, your exercises should have prepared you for holding up your own feet, so just tell the nurses you know what to do, and show them by picking up your legs at the knees. Then at last, when your baby is ready for the world, you are ready to push him out, and if his father is there he'll be ready to receive the being he has helped create.

My husband hadn't cried since he was a baby himself. When his son was born, and he caught the wet little head in the palm of his hand to guide him out through my vagina, emotion poured a glad river of tears over both of us and our son was born into a moment of happiness more complete than any we had yet known.

Shared labour, shared child, shared love, new family.

8

After Birth

Post-Baby Blues

If you feel depressed sometimes in the weeks after having a baby, don't think you are abnormal. It happens to everyone to a greater or lesser degree. You've been through a tremendous physical and emotional experience which is inevitably tiring. This exhaustion is bound to find expression in the days following the elation of birth itself.

The name which doctors give to this period of adjustment is 'puerperium'. It means the time in which you are recovering from pregnancy and labour, returning to normal, and forming a relationship with your baby. Signs of depression are expected, whether it's the occasional teardrop, howls of self-pity, or the serious neurosis or even psychosis that some women suffer from. The technical, physical reason for this highly emotional state can be traced back to the same source as the emotional reactions of pregnancy. There are major readjustments of your hormone balance. During pregnancy the placenta floods your system with female hormones. These are cut off suddenly with the delivery of the placenta,[1] and you are then left in a highly vulnerable condition. The relationship between you and your baby is vital to the baby and vital to you during this time.

Try to avoid any sense of disorientation that may come with the baby being outside you instead of inside you. The first step towards this is doing anything you can to hold your baby the minute he is born. Keep him close to you. Don't let other people make decisions

1. *Dictionary of Pregnancy, Childbirth and Contraception*, by Herbert and Margaret Brant, p. 198, Mayflower, London, 1971.

as to how soon you can touch him, how soon the cord is cut, how soon you can put the child to your breast. Unless there have been complications in labour or delivery, those are your decisions to make.

Leaving the cord to finish pulsating naturally gives the baby the extra advantage of continuing to receive oxygen through his own system, the blood circulating through placenta and cord to him, in the way he has always known it, while his lungs establish their function. The advantage it gives a woman is the feeling that her child is still attached to her. This little creature that has spent the time of its gestation from minute cells to human being within her body, can now be seen and felt. There is no doubt in my mind that emotionally this is an extraordinary and precious few moments in the life of the two. Moments that cannot be repeated. All too soon the umbilical cord will cease to be of any functional use. The baby will breathe independently. There is no longer that tangible link. Until this happens, soften the shock of separation for both of you by establishing contact, by holding him in a way that he can feel your love. The strangeness of leaving you, of leaving the element he knows for the world, the air, that he doesn't, will be less harsh. Allowing the cord to finish working in its own time means that the intimate contact between you will not be severed by sharp untimely scissors, but left to end that cycle naturally.

You can put your baby to your breast immediately after birth, before the cord is cut, if possible. Some babies want to suck right away, especially if there have been no labour drugs to depress that reflex. There won't be milk at this stage, but he will get colostrum, and certainly he will gain reassurance and comfort in finding firm evidence of what he is looking for: you. You are the only familiar being, smell, sense, to a newborn child. Everything else is totally new and probably weird. Giving him the comfort of your breast will help both of you adjust to this different stage of your relationship.

If you get a desperate surge of helplessness in the face of having to care for a new life; if you wonder how on earth you are going to cope with the overwhelming responsibility you have initiated; if you feel intimidated by the fragility of this new human being to whom you gave birth, being able to reach out and touch him or hold him is incredibly reassuring to most women. The more a baby trusts you, the more confidence you will have in yourself; the more familiar the baby is to you, the more confidence you will have in your ability to care for him and the more the baby will trust you. Again, do your utmost to see that physical separation, part of the routine of many hospitals, doesn't hinder the development of your relationship at this sensitive stage.

I found that after the births for which I had prepared, I had very little tension or anxiety during the 'puerperium'. Certainly not the kind of emotional instability or melancholy that could be described as serious post-natal depression. Yet a period of fairly acute depression is considered quite normal by doctors. Gordon Bourne, consultant obstetrician and gynaecologist at St Bartholomew's Hospital, London, observes that 'It is said every new mother should experience "the blues"'. These 'blues' usually last for twelve to twenty-four hours, generally between the third and sixth day after delivery.[1] His explanation for this is that most midwives and doctors consider an attack of the blues virtually essential to relieve tension. My own view is that there is far less likely to be tension if a woman has prepared for her birth in a way that allows her to be conscious for delivery. This way she does not suppress the enormous experience with all its emotional, physical and spiritual implications. If she knows what she is doing during pregnancy, labour and delivery, there is more of a chance of her knowing what she is doing in the period immediately afterwards. Understanding that another huge hormone change is taking place, makes it easier to deal with. Almost all the work I have come across in this area relates post-natal depression to tension. Knowing how to alleviate tension is not something that disappears the moment the baby is born. Awareness is not something which comes and goes so quickly. The things we learn about relaxation during pregnancy apply to the times when we are not pregnant, and most especially to the time immediately after delivery, because if preparation has made both an integrated experience, hopefully that integration will continue.

I feel that Naturebirth not only made a difference to the way I carried and delivered my children, but also to my entire relationship with them outside the womb. I know that depressant drugs sedate and so probably suppress feelings. I think there is a possibility that preparation could help alleviate the distress of women who feel the after-birth period as painful and disturbing for two reasons. It

1. *Pregnancy*, by Gordon Bourne, p. 422, Cassells, London, 1972.

teaches you to experience labour being dependent only on yourself, not on drugs, and it teaches mental and physical awareness and relaxation. These last equip you not only for birth but for life thereafter.

Women who have a bad time giving birth must logically be more likely to harbour resentment afterwards. So there is not only the exhaustion and the hormone upheaval to deal with, but also your own fury. In some women the aftermath is tragic. In Britain, 88,000 women a year have to be treated, usually by a psychiatrist and sedation, for post-natal depression, five times as many women are admitted to mental hospitals in the period shortly after giving birth as normally, and there is no evidence that the incidence of severe post-natal depression has decreased since 1915—although perinatal mortality has been drastically reduced in this time.[1]

On a different level, there is something doctors call 'placenta loss', which means that when you become aware of the fact that there is no longer a child within you, part of you, a sense of loss is experienced, perhaps even loneliness after the intimacy of holding another human being inside your body for nine months. I can relate this loss to my own chilling experience of abortion. However hard we might try to dismiss it intellectually, once pregnant I think we are at some time aware of and sensitive to the life we have initiated, and I found on waking from the anaesthetic there was a sinking drowning feeling of emptiness, of having lost something precious, something part of you. I can understand that 'placenta loss' could be like this, and to some women very terrible.

Most women go through only a brief depression, but for others it persists for much longer than the immediate after-birth period, and in varying degrees. It could last a year, it might develop into incurable psychosis. It seems that no one has worked out a way of dealing with it, because there is no real agreement as to its causes, although out of the ten to twenty thousand women—there seem to be no more precise figures—in Britain who have become psychotic following their confinements in the last ten years, only half have recovered. One of the most significant aspects is that in the few hospitals that have special mother and baby units to cope with post-natal depression without separating mother and child, at least half the patients

1. 'Where Will They Go Tomorrow?' by Lyn Owen, *The Guardian*, London, p. 13, 22nd February, 1973.

had no previous history of psychiatric disturbance.[1] Yet puerperal psychosis as a form of mental illness particular to childbirth is dismissed by some obstetricians despite the fact that 52 per cent of baby-battering cases take place just after a woman has given birth or is pregnant again. There is accepted evidence now that early separation of mother and child can lead to battered babies:

'The battered child syndrome provides the most dramatic evidence of a disorder of mothering ... early separation may be a factor. The formation of close emotional ties may remain permanently incomplete if extended separation occurs.'[2]

Specialists disagree as to the causes and the cures. Some believe there is a genetic element involved, because certain nervous systems appear less able to cope with stress than others. Another view is that the massive upheaval of hormones which takes place during pregnancy and birth may leave an imbalance in some women after they have had the baby. One gynaecologist who believes in this theory is Dr Katherina Dalton.[3] After a survey at the North Middlesex Hospital in England she found that mothers who became postnatally depressed were prone to anxiety at the beginning of pregnancy, but in the later months professed to have 'never felt better'. She believes there is a link between women who are irritable and lethargic around the time of their period, and those who suffer from post-natal depression. Both conditions are due to hormonal fluctuations. Women lacking in progesterone feel depressed. During pregnancy a vast amount of this hormone is generated in our bodies, so that someone with this deficiency would probably feel healthier than usual. After birth they feel the decrease in progesterone which most of us adjust to quite smoothly, as an intense deprivation.[4]

Swedish psychiatrists, Lund and Nilsson, decided from surveys that the endocrine functioning alone could not account for the obsessional and sometimes psychotic states of some women. They found the most susceptible women are unmarried mothers, those

1. 'Where Will They Go Tomorrow?', by Lyn Owen, *The Guardian*, London, p. 13, 22nd February, 1973.
2. See Marshall Klaus, M.D., 'Human Behavior at the first Contact with Her Young', *Pediatrics*, 46: 187–92, U.S.A. *Also* 'Maternal Attachment: Importance of the First Post-Partum Days', *New England Journal of Medicine*, 286: 460–3, 1970.
3. *The Menstrual Cycle*, by Katherina Dalton, London, 1969.
4. *Pregnancy*, by Gordon Bourne, p. 447, Cassells, London, 1972.

with insecurities arising from their own childhoods, and professional women in conflict with the traditional female role.

Birth trauma is accentuated by fear and tension. Women who approach childbirth in a state of extreme anxiety can slow down their own labours, by bracing against contractions out of fear, so causing muscular spasm which prevents the cervix from dilating. This kind of anxiety continues to be felt after birth, and there does seem to be some connection between *long* labours and extreme depression.

One reason for this kind of tension could be the unfamiliar surroundings of a hospital. Almost all surveys indicate that hospital deliveries produce more post-natal depression than home deliveries. In Wales, for instance, a medical survey showed 65 per cent of mothers were affected by depression in hospital, and only 19 per cent at home.[1] I think all possible reasons for evidence like this should be examined, especially since some women either want to kill their babies or are afraid they will, and more than half of the cases of baby-battering take place when the mother has just given birth or is pregnant again.[1]

There is obviously no easy answer either to the reasons or the cures. The medical establishment suggest only cures, as far as I can see: drugs, hormone treatment, psychotherapy or mental institutions. After the event. My instinct is to resort to common sense, by attempting prevention first.

Perhaps our attitude to birth and ability to relate to our children afterwards may make a difference to the degree in which we suffer depression. The light and shade of the entire experience of birth may influence this. Perhaps it is natural to feel certain resentment at the discomfort of labour, and indeed pregnancy, only we bury it, especially, I would think, if the labour is heavily sedated, so it doesn't surface until after the baby is born.

A quick solution is to tell someone to admit it, as soon as you feel it stirring, so that it doesn't build into a violent emotion you cannot control. More important, I believe the whole concept of preparing for birth should help reduce such tensions. Since I also think sedating drugs have a depressing effect emotionally as well as physically, knowing how to avoid suppressing the sensations of

1. Both references from *Nova*, June 1973, pp. 56–7, and *The Guardian*, London, p. 13, 22nd February, 1973.

giving birth by avoiding deep sedation might allow feelings of all kinds to be expressed as they happen. In that case, after delivery a woman is less likely to lash herself out of a sense of repression by exploding in anger at the creature who apparently caused it all.

If being institutionalized to have your baby upsets you, and the association between hospitals, disease, patients and death often does confuse a woman's sense of identity—then consider a home delivery. Or if that isn't possible, remember that you can transform hospital space. Try having things around you that remind you of home. It could be flowers, candles, pictures, books, scent, a pretty bed cover, a plant, photographs of the people you love, little boxes or trinkets that have some special meaning. Encourage those closest to you to visit often, so you don't lose contact with the outside world, especially your man, or your other children.

Most important of all, don't lose contact with your baby. This is when you learn to know your child as an individual. The umbilical cord has been cut, but that doesn't have to mean the intense bond between you is severed. It takes time and peace to adjust to the change, but it is simply a change in the nature of the bond, not an end to it.

Too often separation is the name of the game of medical science. Separation in the name of science, medicine, hygiene, routine, or anything other than safety, is a cut, break, scission, disruption, corruption, irreparable breach, even dismemberment. The wound may never be healed if undertaken too crudely. The scissor cutting the cord through which life blood flows is a cold blade. The starch of a nurse's apron is stiff where a naked breast is soft. A glass cage and tubes are seldom better than love or warmer than skin. A clean cot is colder than a human body. Sugar and water are thin nourishment against the richness of colostrum which, springing from the nipple before the milk comes through, gives our newborn the immunity we have ourselves—up to a year's protection from even the common cold. Hearts should beat together while they can.

Breastfeeding

This is an enormous subject, on which there is now a vast amount of research being undertaken. The fashion for breastfeeding and for bottle feeding has swung backwards and forwards as each method competed for popularity during the last few years. Bottle feeding offered freedom to women who did not want to be tied to their babies by the nipple. Yet bottle feeding seemed to be leading to fat babies and fat babies to fat adults. All sorts of defects were found in the artificial formulae, women made mistakes in concocting the bottle milk, it was discovered that babies were actually dying from dehydration which could be traced to over-feeding from the bottle.

I cannot undertake a detailed analysis of the advantages and disadvantages of breastfeeding in this book because the subject ranges too far, and I would feel irresponsible presenting this brief discussion as anything but that, but I must bring it up in order that women who are preparing for birth may also know something of the facts of afterbirth before the event.

Breastfeeding is one way of maintaining close contact with your baby. It is also a way of ensuring that he stays beside you if you are in hospital. A baby is less a part of the routine when his feeding schedule is up to you. If he is being fed by a nurse through a bottle with dozens of other children, it's understandable for the nurses to want to set a time and a place for the mass feeds that have nothing to do with you, because very often it does have nothing to do with you. If you yourself are feeding him by bottle, it is still easier for the length and the times of the feeds to be regulated by the hospital. If you breastfeed on demand, it is clearly up to you when you do it and for how long.

I have always enjoyed breastfeeding and found it a peaceful and comforting time. Quite apart from the fact that the baby's sucking helps the uterus contract back to its normal size more quickly, I love the sensual contact with this tiny newborn creature, it gives me a sense of belonging to the child and the child to me. Perhaps it is possessive, but this particular kind of possessiveness, which may have something to do with making up for placenta loss, doesn't last long, and creates a kind of hallowed circle around the two of you that is particular to that time and that act.

I know many women are put off by the sexuality of the child's mouth sucking on the nipple, and that sometimes fathers can find it sexually disturbing and feel jealous. There may well be a difference in feeding a male child and a female child; it is not something I can tell from experience, since I have never borne a girl. To me such inhibitions are understandable, and I am sure it would be quite wrong to nurse your child if you find it disturbing, or an interference in your marital relationship. Babies seem to sense things extraordinarily quickly, and it could possibly be harmful to the child if you try to nurse against your own desires. If you have decided not to breastfeed, as the majority of women do today, don't feel guilty about it. Each woman and each child is biologically and psychologically different, so it is always a question of individual choice, and guilt has no place in these kinds of decisions.

However, do resist the kind of social pressures which could lead you to feel you were doing something slightly unattractive, tasteless, or harmful to the baby, if you do want to breastfeed. Don't allow your own maternal instincts to be squashed by hospital regime, the prudish disapproval of bodily contact, any insistence by family or neighbours that it is 'beneath' someone like you to revert to the primitive in such a way, the bombardment of advertising campaigns for artificial milk and baby foods proclaimed more natural than the natural and certainly more beneficial to the baby. Not to mention the manufacturers. Remember that routine is not impenetrable, sensuality is less confusing than inhibited response, class consciousness is utterly meaningless in the face of developing a new relationship, and the artificial seldom adequately replaces the natural.

I feel bound to encourage women to breastfeed if they can, not only because I know the closeness and warmth it can generate between you and your child in this the earliest part of your relationship with one another, but because there is medical evidence that it is healthier for the child.

Dr Marshall H. Klaus, neonatologist, professor of pediatrics and director of nurseries at Case Western University in America, has found that breastfed babies are less likely to become constipated or contract skin disorders and respiratory infections. They also have seven times fewer allergies, and can handle foreign proteins more easily.[1]

They are protected from obesity as well as disease, because it is so easy to overfeed with bottle formulas, and there are a worrying number of nutritional ailments caused by feeds that are made up incorrectly.[2] Different brands of artificial milk have different

1. 'Giving Birth', by Melissa Sones, *Ramparts*, p. 53, September 1974.
2. 'Why Some Babies Don't Sleep', by Martin Richards, Judith Bernal, *New Society*, p. 510, 28th February, 1974.

compositions, and where one will suit one baby, it may not another, just as breastfeeding may suit one woman and for others it could be a nightmare.

We lead completely different lives today from those of the primitive women for whom breastfeeding was the only way to nourish their children. The structure of our society separates us from our children far more, so that instead of being in more or less continuous contact with them, day and night, the normal procedure is to separate infant and mother at birth and for that separation to continue. To breast-feed you have to have your baby with you most of the time. You are the only one who can give him sustenance. Anyone can give a baby a bottle. The convenience of it sounds seductive to some women, women who are perhaps unaware of how easy it is simply to unbutton your shirt and put your baby to your breast. I found it far more complicated to sterilize bottles and teats every day, warm the milk to the right temperature, and make sure the measurement of artificial milk to water is absolutely correct. Above everything, the contact between woman and child is less intimate and personal.

As in all matters of choice, it is invaluable to have at hand as much information as is available and, while I cannot quite give you that, I can point out some of the advantages to breastfeeding now being discovered in research. The subject is vast and controversial, so this is only a guide, not a complete assessment of the entire picture.

For instance, breastfed babies are less vulnerable to infection generally, but particularly in the case of gastro-enteritis,[1] an illness that small babies can contract quite easily. Iron-binding proteins in human milk provide resistance to infection,[2] and there is evidence of protection against septicaemia (blood poisoning),[3] plus immunity to polio can be transferred in breast milk[4] and the incidence of dental troubles and allergies are definitely lower in breastfed babies.[5]

I have already remarked how complicated it can be to sterilize all the bottle equipment for formula feeding, but apparently even the

1. Bullen, C. L. and Wills, A. T.: 'Resistance of the Breastfed Infant to Gastroenteritis', *British Medical Journal*, 3: 338, 1971.
2. Bullen, J. J., Rogers, H. J., and Leigh, L.: *British Medical Journal*, 1:69, 1972.
3. J. Winberg and G. Wesser, *The Lancet*, 1: 109, 1971.
4. Katz, M. and Plotkin, S. A.: 'Oral polio immunization of the newborn infant', *Journal of Pediatrics*, 73: 267, 1968.
5. Gloser, J.: 'The Dietary Prophylaxis of Allergic Disease in Infancy', *Journal of Asthma Research*, 3: 199, 1966.

methods used for sterilization can lead to contamination of the milk.[1] If overconcentrated feeds are given, as is sometimes encouraged by professional advice and the advertising of manufacturers, babies then need extra water to cope with the solidity of the feed and the dehydration that results. Few women are taught to recognize that a baby might be crying from thirst rather than hunger. It is possible that the carbohydrates present in artificial milk may be habit-forming and increase later consumption of sugars and all the risks of obesity that go with that.

Dr Peter Andrews, a British Home Office pathologist, states that the dehydration from overstrong baby food might be a contributing factor in cot deaths. If the baby has a mild infection, then sweats in his cot, his body might be too dried out to cope. In a study of fifty-four cot deaths,[2] Dr Andrews found that fifty-two of the babies showed signs of dehydration, and their waste products and stomach contents suggested that the relatively high salt content of the feeds, compared with mother's milk, caused the dehydration. By January 1976 statistics showed that three thousand cot deaths a year were due to causes related to dehydration from artificial baby foods.

There are two points which seem to me to be particularly significant. One is that dangerously high levels of lead (intake 900 micrograms a day) have been found in tinned formulas in America,[3] and the other is that there appears to be less risk of a baby dying in his cot when he is being fed from the breast.

Both Britain and America have far more bottle-fed than breastfed babies—a recent survey of England and Wales showed that only 6 per cent of babies more than twelve weeks old were breastfed—but there does seem to be a case either for re-examining the make-up of the formulas, or encouraging more women to feed their babies themselves. This could be done by giving them more information as they become pregnant, and by helping them overcome whatever psychological, emotional, sexual or even social objections they may have against nursing from the breast.

1. Anderson, J. A. D. and Catherer, A.: *British Medical Journal*, 1: 20, 1970.
2. Research by Dr Peter Andrews, published in *Medicine, Science and the Law*, 1975.
3. Doherty, G. A., Gates, A. H., and Sewell, C. E.: 'Methyl-mercury transmission via sucking in mouse and man'. In Kretchner, N. and Rossi, E. (eds), *Milk and Lactation*, Basel, Karger, in press.

POSTSCRIPT

A Letter to Sara

Sara being with me right through Orion's labour and the moment of birth, was so moving and rewarding in all the shades and levels of the experience that she asked me to write her a letter afterwards. She asked for a birth report, the story of the birth and my feelings, assessing how much the preparation had affected me and the course of labour. The idea grew into this book.

So here I will print the letter I sent to Sara after Orion was born. Her first birth report. I have left in all the obvious emotional overtones because it was simply how I felt. I was writing to her about a profound experience so nearly devoid of fear and pain that the letter is beyond logic, intellect, reason or objectivity. Take it for what it is. The account of an act of love.

From Danaë to Sara
London—January 1971

Dear Sara,

Spring this year is childbirth.

Orion was born, and I was absolutely aware. I'm writing to thank you for helping me make the trip.

You taught me to breathe, and through controlling each breath during contractions, I could control pain. I didn't get lost in that pain swamp I remember from my eldest son's birth, and I think that's the secret of the method you teach, you don't get lost. It's vital that people realize that your head can guide your body through anything, even the extremes of childbirth. Lucky I met you when I did, because you marched through fear and forced me to discipline my head in a way I would never have thought possible, if I hadn't just done it.

Instead of drowning, I learnt how to swim—an acceptable analogy because physical agony of that nature works like a tidal wave. The breaking pattern is a mental surf-board to heave yourself onto and ride out the wave. It's when you get swamped that fear reduces you to a gibbering wreck and all you can think of is why don't they get the strongest drug in the whole fucking hospital and shove it into your body to stop this thing that's tearing you apart. It's ignorance and fear that makes you feel you are dying, that blinds you to the fact that this is a birth process, that panics you out of the miracle into the nightmare. I know, because I went through that with my first child.

But with the second it was your discipline, Mrs Harrison, making me sit on the floor like a rag doll, feeling self-conscious and foolish, legs spread, breathing to the pattern on those weird diagrams—level A, B, C, and D—each breath getting more and more shallow to cope with the make-believe muscle-contractions, forcing me to stay there while we went through the charade again and again, when all I wanted to do was lie around—lazy, not thinking about the inevitable. Push it away, I figured, it won't really happen if I don't think about it.

But you made me think about it, talk about it, dream about it, jump right into the middle of the realization of birth as the ultimate creative act, with receptivity the fundamental link between two life forces. Your practical daily discipline showed me that fear was the devil—not very heavily disguised—and confidence, which somehow or other you helped me achieve, the guardian angel.

I started to do exercises much later than normally advised. Most people start in the sixth month of pregnancy, I was eight months when we began, so it was a concentrated onslaught between the first controlled breath and Orion's birth cry.

I read Erna Wright's book, *The New Childbirth*. I listened to you tell me you made it through a difficult birth with your fourth child without drugs, and that it was still the most exhilarating experience of all. You turned me on to the possibilities of my own power to deal with pain, but I didn't really believe it until I was in the labour room, wrecked physically, but soaring mentally.

Up until the time we reached the hospital, I was hard to convince I was actually in labour. We began timing the contractions at about

6 p.m. but I was still prancing round the house, getting supper for the eight-year-old, telling myself those occasional flashes were imagination, unable to believe the process had begun, because I didn't feel nervous. I felt excited, didn't feel apprehension, it was anticipation.

I'd got ready most of the things needed to take to the hospital for the baby and myself. After I'd rung you, and then the hospital, and matron had told me to be there in an hour, I speeded up and packed the last of the necessary things, including that natural sponge which helped immeasurably during heavy labour when your lips get so unbearably dry from the open-mouthed breathing.

On reflection it was amazing the hospital allowed in not only you, but two of my dearest friends, whose energy buoyed me up through those long hours between going into the labour room at 9 p.m., and Orion's birth at 1.09 a.m. the next morning. Receptivity applies on every level to a woman so close to giving birth. All the love that was coming from the three of you fed me extra strength when most needed.

Although I could feel the midwife approved of my efforts to do without the respite of painkillers, she treated me rather as though I were a good hockey player whom the team expected to keep going regardless of obstacles. I became less and less aware of the nurses, and even the doctor, as time wore on and my body wore out. I felt rather than saw the three of you, knowing that if at any point I couldn't cope you'd be there to tell me I could.

The most important thing you taught me, both before and during the birth, was that you don't need drugs to go through pain and come out on the other side. You can do it alone. And it is quite a journey. I was entirely aware of the pain, and still remember, so clear was each facet of the experience, its every trap and sharp edge, remember feeling its teeth in my abdomen, watching it ebb and flow with my invisible breath, running with it up and down the cracks on the labour room ceiling, plunging in and out of it as the contractions plunged in and out of me, pulling it this way and that as the child pulled at my stomach and pelvic muscles, dancing with it along the corridors of my own childhood, evoked by that ridiculous song—D'Ye Ken John Peel—you insisted I learn, so that mouthing it and tapping out the rhythm with my fingers on the bed would distract me from the worst of the struggle—'transition', that phase before the baby's head is far enough down the birth channel to push and the mother's body is stretched almost beyond the limits of endurance—but not quite. Your hovering presence then reminded me there's no such thing as beyond the limit of endurance if you tell yourself there's no such thing. And there wasn't. The diagrams flashed black and white in front of my eyes. I didn't do it right all the time, but when I didn't you could see the loss of control and nudged me back on top again with a sharp word, so I rode it, controlled its effect, psychic and physical, so I didn't freak out, so I was together enough to talk to the three of you, who seemed as exhilarated as I, all of us caught in that crystal prism of pure energy that was in fact the four of us giving birth, through my body, to a new life. That happening the books call a miracle and for which I have no words that do more than approximately convey its truth. All I can tell you is that at the moment of birth—on that third push when the nurse said 'Your baby's coming—look!' and I called out for the first time during the whole labour (I can hear the cry now, but maybe it wasn't a cry, it was a grunt or a groan, a sound wrenched out like the involuntary ecstatic gasp of orgasm) when my son shot out like a small wet cannonball, his yelling joining mine—the experience transcended words.

I touched him and knew, absolutely, that I could do it again. Thank you for showing me how.

Danaë

The foundations for life and love are laid before birth. Feel conception's miraculous dance; watch the progress of gestation; be in awe of the process of birth; understand the fundamental truth that magic lies in our union with nature, not in the struggle against it. There is strength in awareness that comes from seeing all sides, knowing weakness, and moving on. Preparation is a weapon and a gift. Let it be our gift to the children of the future.

Perhaps, simply, natural birth followed through with love may take the pain from being born and be the basis of a loving family. Not the family of laws and mores, documents and dictatorship, but the family of freedom. Preparation may help us redefine that lost identity. It is we who want children who must make the change.

Wilhelm Reich said: 'The natural family is based on love'. I am looking for a way for the natural family to survive.

A POEM TO MY HUSBAND

If you have been alone, there is a subtle change
in the quality of life shared in love;
the difference between cloud and mist, shade and shadow;
sharing birth is the same kind of poem.
Catch it if you can.

Acknowledgement and Thanks to:

Sara Harrison, without whom I might never have learned about prepared childbirth and the enlightenment it can bring; Ronnie Laing whose work in psychiatry is continually improving birth conditions and feeding me with information; Andre Schiffrin, Milly Daniel and Peter Grose who kept faith in my writing and kept me to it; Sir Robert Lusty whose idea it was that I forsake the piles of nappies for a typewriter to get on paper the depths of my feelings; The National Childbirth Trust which provides so many women with the impetus to fend off technology and experience natural birth; Elizabeth Bing whose helpful comments undoubtedly made this book more readable for American women; Suzanne Arms who burst into our lives just before *Naturebirth* was published and helped me along with encouragement and support, having herself been through the experience of writing a book on birth; Rachel Monsarrat whose enthusiasm and objectivity as an editor made that final stage so much less isolated; Dr John Bradshaw who cast his meticulous eye over the medical information to make sure there were no flaws, and Dr Robert Lefever who spent long night hours presenting the view of enlightened doctors; John Damonte, from whom I learned so much about homoeopathy; Ann Warren-Davis, medical herbalist, who checked all the information on healing herbs; Harriet Bloomer whose careful research enabled me to double check the most controversial references; Helen Brew who reinforced my belief in the damage caused by separating infants from their mothers at birth; my dear friends, Dari and Karen, the Thunderthigh songbirds, who forsook their music for the keys of a typewriter at deadline crisis when, without their help, both book and babies might have been neglected; and all the men and women who were so moved by preparing through pregnancy for the impact of watching their children being born, that they prompted me to report the experiences of all of us who have shared in this so that others may come to believe as I do in the power and precision of nature in birth.

APPENDIX I

Physical Exercises

Exercises for muscle dissociation, muscle tone and relaxation, and exercises for breathing can all begin after about the sixteenth week of pregnancy, as long as your doctor approves and there is no complication in the pregnancy which might preclude physical exertion.

Conscious Muscle Control

One of the unexpected things about labour which makes it so peculiarly difficult to handle is the strangeness of feeling one set of muscles at work independently from the rest of the body. It will not feel so odd if we have experienced something similar before we go into labour. So it is important to simulate this before labour begins. It accustoms you to the sensation and gives you a clue as to how to cope with it.

The following physical exercises have been put together to give you an idea of the type of feeling created by the uterus contracting while the rest of your body is kept as relaxed as possible. This is the secret of a flowing labour. Your body is not hindering the work of your womb. The baby is being helped by you, not held back.

Conscious separation of one set of muscles from another shows you how the uterine muscles can be working while the rest of your body is relaxed: to understand first the difference between a tense and a relaxed set of muscles, take very basic and simple exercises.

If you raise one arm from the elbow, tighten the fist, clench it really hard, and then let go, you should be really *feeling* the difference as the tenseness leaves the arm, wrist, hand, and fingers. Doing it

247

several times will accustom you to being aware of the sensation, so that you can pick up on it if it happens to your body during the normal course of the day—which of course it does often, especially under city life pressure. Most people tense and contract if shocked—when you just miss another car when you're driving—when a kid rushes across the road—when you drop a tray full of glasses. Feel what is happening to you inside, and then breathe out, let go, relax. It really helps.

A good, but rather extreme, way of understanding how to locate and then dissociate from the kind of tension created by clenched muscles, is by one person doing a 'Chinese burn' or 'Indian torture' on the other.

Exercise I

One person takes the loose skin of another's arm, encircling it with two hands twisting in opposite directions. When the person being tortured feels the pain, she gasps in shock. When this is done to you, feel yourself tighten up against what's happening to the arm. Consciously relax and breathe out. This not only loosens your tension and minimizes your reaction to it, but it also gets rid of that sudden fear.

A less violent and perhaps more precise way of getting used to the difference between tenseness and relaxation is as follows:

Exercise II

Sit on the floor comfortably, with your back well supported by cushions propped up against a wall, or something solid and upright like a sofa or armchair. Think carefully about each group of muscles in your body. Tighten them separately and then let go. Work up from your toes, through your feet, calves, thighs, stomach, chest, neck etc., till you reach your head. Try to make sure there's someone else watching because they can actually see the difference in what is happening to your muscles.

Exercises consciously to relax face and associated muscles. Just before doing the breathing practice, or after a long hard day, try this ·

Exercise I

Purse your lips very tight as though screwing them together. Let go very gently. Then clench your jaw as you would to bite through a piece of steel, and let go very gently. Frown so hard that you're scowling, and then slowly let your forehead uncrease to its normal velvet smoothness.

Sticking your tongue out as far as it can possibly go will relax it. Pressing your neck hard back against cushions and then letting go slowly will relax a part of you which probably gets very tired from holding your head up all day, but which we forget about most of the time. Remember to massage your neck with cream afterwards, especially if you do these exercises at night, or after a bath. The more relaxed the muscles the more absorbent the skin. And it's soothing too.

Exercise II

Consciously shrug your shoulders up around your neck as high as they'll go. Remember what you did at school when you wanted to be rude to the teacher but didn't dare speak? That's it. The sullen shrug. Heave them up, and then let them go slowly. Heave them up, and let them go.

Note: When you are doing these exercises at home it is usually best to make them the last thing you do before going to bed at night. That way you're all set to relax completely afterwards, either in a hot bath or a warm bed.

Toning Exercises

In order to keep your figure in trim, and ready to shape up as quickly as possible after the baby is born, you need to make sure that the *abdominal wall*, which is continually slowly stretching to accommodate and hold the baby, is supple enough to slip back into firm shape after the birth. The following exercises should help:

Exercise

Lie flat on the floor (or the bath, or the bed, depending where you choose to do it), knees bent upwards, feet flat. Put your hands on your belly, feel the shape of the baby, and then, tightening the stomach muscles slowly, try sort of pulling the baby down gently towards your backbone with your own muscles. Then relax. Practise this about ten times.

The next exercise is for toning up the internal muscles, the *pelvic floor*, which is the area of muscles between the pelvic bones around and deep inside the vagina. The pelvis is that bony area of you around the hips which holds in bladder, tubes, ovaries, rectum, part of the bowels and, of course, the baby. The pelvic floor is the area of internal muscles around the lower pelvic bones. A man's is shaped like a triangle. A woman's, when she isn't pregnant, is the shape and size of a pear. This is one of the best exercises for feeling the link between correct breathing and working with a set of muscles that are, to many people, unfamiliar. You can learn to feel and manipulate the muscles of the vagina and rectum internally, and should, since they are the muscles most under the strain during pregnancy and birth. You have one ring of muscles round your anus and another set around your vagina; if not used they can get like an old elastic band—stretched and useless—not strong enough to spring back into shape after they've been pulled. You need to know how to distinguish between the two rings of muscles, because when you are having the baby you don't want to be pushing him out with your anal muscles, but those in your vagina and, unless you have tried to separate the two sets consciously, it is hard to then do so in labour. First you learn to dissociate, and so really feel the two sets of muscles separately, then you learn how to keep the whole area in tone.

Exercise 1

Try to keep your anus relaxed while you pull in your vagina, and your vagina relaxed while you pull in your anal passage muscles, as if you needed to shit but you have to hold it in. One way of checking out the accuracy of what you are doing is to practise using the different sets of muscles while on the lavatory. If you can stop the flow while taking a pee you are using your vaginal muscles correctly. Imagine putting, or actually put, your fingers into your vagina to test whether the muscles are working strongly. If you can feel the squeeze then you're all right.

People get very used to holding themselves in down there. And so much of the idea of the pain in having a baby is involved in that area that it is vital to know the difference between how it is when contracted and tight, and how it is when relaxed. Another way to practise, and be aware of using these vaginal muscles, is when you are making love. Hold your man inside you as long as you can, let him feel the suction of you clasping and letting go. As with most of the exercises for this birth preparation, it helps your sex life too.

The next step is to pull up both sets of muscles together. Now you are using the *whole of the pelvic floor*. Once you've tightened anal and vaginal muscles, pull them up, let go very slowly, and then relax.

To really feel the second pelvic floor exercise, try this:

Exercise II

Imagine your pelvic floor is like a department store lift and you are going to take it up to different levels. No other muscles should come into play except those around the vagina and anus. Put your hand on your pubis, feel the muscles inside, feel your vagina round to your anus. That's the whole area we're dealing with. Now pull in and upwards. It's a lift. Take it up to the first floor, then the second floor, and then the third floor and the fourth floor. Hold it. Now let it down one floor, then another floor, then the next floor, and you've reached the ground level. Now push it down to the basement and bring it back up again to where it should be: ground level.

A good tip to remember all through pregnancy is when you have to get up from lying on your back or sitting on the floor, roll onto your stomach first, then get up on all fours like a bear, before you finally heave yourself into standing position. It takes the strain off muscles if you get them ready for movement first.

Here's another tip—this time for backache—the bane of my pregnant life. Play the bear again. Get on all fours. Allow your spine to sink towards the floor like a sagging mattress but leave your bottom in the air like a duck with its head among the pond weeds. Then draw up your stomach and pull in your tail. Hold it for a moment or two, then slowly let go. Do it about six times. It will relieve strain and make your spine more supple.

Breathing

All the breathing exercises have been worked out so the body can be relaxed. We learn mind and body consciousness because improving sensory awareness is an important part of preparing ourselves for childbirth—it is easier to stay in control of something you understand. Each exercise calls for a completely slack mouth, which in turn ensures the relaxation of your vagina. Keeping your mouth open is a vital point of the breathing. You breathe in through your nose and out through your mouth, but your lips rest slightly apart all the time.

The following charts illustrate a technique for practising relaxation through altering levels of breathing throughout labour. Each chart correlates to the cycle of one hypothetical contraction. During practice you can shorten the length of time between early, mild, contractions, for which level A breathing is used, for the sake of time and convenience. Timing on the charts is inevitably approximate since the pace of each labour will vary. Contractions can be simulated by a partner pinching tender skin on the mother, so showing how primary pain can be handled through conscious controlled breathing. Keeping palms upturned during exercises is a good way to keep a check on overall relaxation.

BREATHING LEVELS.

Breathing starts deeply in level A and becomes progressively shallower as levels B, C and D, move up from the diaphragm to the throat, in relation to the increased intensity of contractions as labour progresses.

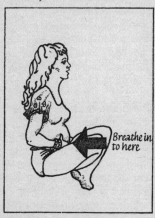

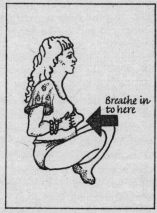

A Deep breath inflating the diaphragm.

B Slightly more shallow breath in to level of the lower ribcage.

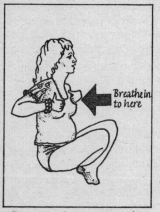

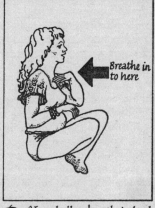

C Shallow breath to level of the breastbone.

D Very shallow breath to level of the collarbone.

You can start off by feeling the different levels from which your breathing will come. Just touch your body with your fingertips. For the first level, the deep breathing, put your fingers just below your ribcage in the area between the last ribs and the beginning of your stomach muscles, which is called the diaphragm. Breathe in through your nose with your mouth closed and you will find you have to expand your chest as much as you can. The diaphragm moves downward and outward with this in-breath and you can see your fingers being pushed out as the diaphragm becomes inflated. As you breathe out through your mouth, feel the muscles of the diaphragm move up and in again with the air being pushed out, and so your fingers go in again.

For the next level, move your fingertips up to the lower ribcage, and with your mouth open breathe in and out, the breath a little more shallow than before, to match the stronger contraction. Now move your fingers to the level of your breastbone and take the breathing from there. The fourth level is way up in your chest, almost to the throat, and there is practically no effort at all. The air needed by the body flows gently in and out, and rather than controlling it at this level, you have a rhythm, or song, on which to concentrate so that very shallow breathing takes care of itself.

Now let's think about dealing with the progressively stronger contractions in the first part of labour.

Breathing Exercises

For the early stages you use level A, the deepest breathing, just an in-breath through the nose and out-breath exhaled from the mouth. There are such mild contractions at the beginning that until your waters break, you will be able to deal with them walking about the house, cooking dinner, having a bath, or simply lying in bed getting some rest before going to the hospital.

First choose a spot on the wall or a picture on which to focus your eyes. Your eyes need to move around a shape so they don't become fixed and static. Anything in your body that you let become wooden is going against the natural flow. Any tightening or stiffening is holding back. Make sure the pattern you'll follow with your eyes is high enough for your head to resist drooping. Eyelids have to be open to keep yourself alert and in touch. Before you start the breathing, check round your body for relaxation, taking one set of muscles at a time, feeling everything loose. Keep your palms up to ensure loose, relaxed hands as they rest on the floor beside you.

Level A is just breathing in through the nose and out through the mouth regularly, as in basic yoga breathing. You take the breath in, hold it right down below your diaphragm in the space between your stomach muscles and your ribcage, then blow out through your mouth so that it feels as though the breath is pushed up and out from below your diaphragm. You can actually see and feel your stomach moving in and out with this breathing, the deepest you will be doing during labour—and incidentally the way we should breathe all the time, but usually don't. It ensures maximum oxygen to the lungs and helps your entire body relax. The cervix is now beginning to get thinner, in readiness for dilation, which is when the mouth of the womb draws back slowly for the baby's head to emerge.

Level B means a move up a little—it works from the lower ribcage rather than the space between ribcage and belly. You breathe in through your nose and out through your mouth in the same way as level A, but at a more shallow level, and your mouth should be open all the time. If you put the tip of your tongue on the roof of your mouth, it helps keep your mouth soft and supple, marks the distance there should be between your open lips, and keeps them moist. At this time the first stage of labour is established and the cervix begins dilation.

Level C is definitely more shallow than the first two. Its movement originates around the breastbone, way above the ribcage, and the rhythm is faster and lighter. I found it the most useful of all during labour while the cervix was still dilating. I could deal with strong contractions in this level, and still feel I had level D in hand for any ultimate emergencies. It gave me a psychological lift as well as being the easiest to remember. You just breathe in lightly and when you push the breath out you actually say 'out', or, to exaggerate (which helps you remember what you're doing), say 'hout' 'hout'. Accentuating the invisible 'h' makes sure you're really pushing it and helps you hold the correct level. There's something, too, about saying it aloud, which keeps you in touch with your own rhythm. In the later stages of labour I say it resoundingly, so that it comes out almost as a groan. The more moans and groans you make the better. Labour isn't the time for self-consciousness and the more noises you let out the less you're holding in.

Level D is for dealing with the strongest contractions, those which lead up to 'transition', that part of labour when you feel you want to push but there is some reason why you should not. Until that point, labour moves from mild, irregular contractions which last about thirty seconds and come about every thirty minutes, to very strong contractions as the cervix is reaching full dilation which can last up to a minute or more with only a couple of minutes in between. Level D helps with the strongest of the strong, and is where the mind-prevention technique comes into its own. In order to regulate your breathing to as shallow a level as possible, you learn a song by heart, or recall one from childhood memories, the rhythm and verse of which come easily to mind. When the time comes to move up from level C, because saying 'hout, hout' just isn't quite enough to take you over the contraction, you change gear into level D and begin to mouth the words of the song while at the same time tapping out its rhythm with the fingers of one hand.

The idea is that with your mouth open and tongue loosely relaxed, as it is when you are whispering the words of a song, you can breathe without any extra effort and your chest and shoulders are completely relaxed. The air needed by you and the baby will flow gently in and out with the rhythm of the song, without your having to concentrate on anything other than the words.

Having a precise pattern of words and timing to concentrate on relaxes your body and relieves your mind of any effort but that of being inside the song in your head. There's no time left to register discomfort or to wail about it. Your mind dissociates from the stress of your body. You don't interrupt the efficiency and rhythm of these very strong contractions which are pushing your child out of the womb and bringing you to the point of delivery. It's the most difficult time to relax, and the most vital. Any withdrawing or unconscious contraction now would slow things up and work against the dilation of the cervix.

I found that by tapping out the rhythm and mouthing the words, my imagination would run away with the song images. If you know yoga and want to use a mantra, do so—the principle is the same. You are able to accept more feeling if your mind is in a place which pays no heed to stress.

To give you an idea of how to move from one level to another, depending on the length and strength of contractions, imagine that you have a contraction grabbing at your belly. As it starts you can deal with it in level A, but not for long. A is really for the very beginning of labour when contractions last only a few seconds and can have a long time between them. As the contractions get stronger, longer and more frequent, you move up to B, then C, and as you're breathing 'hout hout', you realize that the intensity is forcing you to do something else. So now you ease into your favourite song. It is important to have a song that you know well, because then you don't have to bother your head with whether or not you can remember the words—they're just stashed away in your memory cells ready to pop out as you open the door. Anything from 'Honky Tonk Woman' to a lullaby will do. If your preference is for Stone hard rock then that's what you'll get into on the delivery bed. If you like gentle folk music, then let that be your distraction. Whatever your personal taste in music, let it flow through you, and don't worry about letting others in on the secret.

Make sure you mouth the song emphatically, this loosens the face muscles and is more important than actually hearing yourself sing. The 'conductor' of the preparation group should check round all the time to see that eyes aren't glazing, face muscles are relaxed and no worried frowns are creasing the brows.

Now that you know the mechanics of the breathing, try practising with one person reading out instructions as he or she times each contraction. The person doing this 'conducting' of the practice should start off by saying 'Contractions start now', and then, noting the approximate length of time each contraction should take (indicated in the following charts), start off in level A, observe how each woman is breathing and how relaxed she is, then finish off the pretend contraction by saying 'It's gone' so everyone knows when to finish and take a deep cleansing breath before starting on the next one.

The timing need not be rigid, all times are approximate and all labours different. This is just for practice—not a rule to be obeyed.

1. *Weak contractions—deep breathing*

Level A breathing only, for the duration of thirty seconds, one cleansing breath and three resting breaths between simulated contractions. (These resting breaths are for practice. During early labour the interval will probably be much longer than this.)

Go through it several times without changing levels, with the conductor saying 'Contraction starts now', and, after about thirty seconds, 'Contraction ends now'.

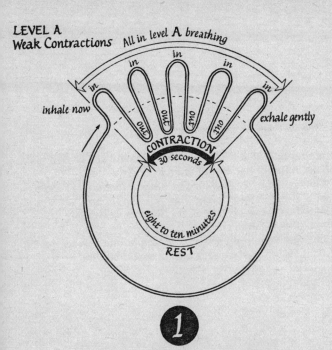

All in level A breathing

in · in · in · in · in

inhale now · out · out · out · exhale gently

CONTRACTION
30 seconds

eight to ten minutes

REST

①

DEEP BREATHING

For use during mild contractions in very early labour, when the thinning of the cervix begins.

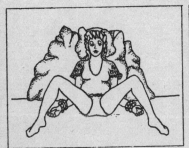
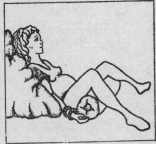

A Take in a deep breath through your nose, inflating your diaphragm. As you let go, exhale through your mouth.

2. *Medium contractions—medium breathing*

Start with level A breathing, go up to level B and down again to level A for the duration of one minute.

Go through it like this: conductor says, 'Contraction starts now' after four breaths in level A, say: 'Getting stronger' after four breaths in level B, say: 'Getting weaker' after four breaths in level A, say: 'It's gone' one cleansing breath and three resting breaths between contractions (as before, the resting breaths are for practice, there will be a longer interval during labour).

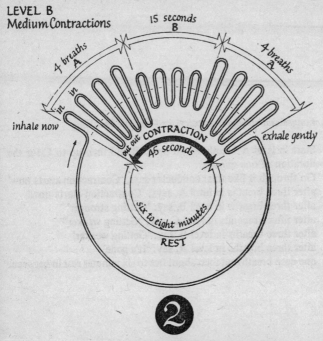

LEVEL B
Medium Contractions

15 seconds
B

4 breaths A

4 breaths A

in

out CONTRACTION

inhale now

exhale gently

45 seconds

six to eight minutes

REST

② MEDIUM BREATHING

For use during the slightly longer and stronger contractions that develop as the first stage of labour is established and the cervix begins to dilate.

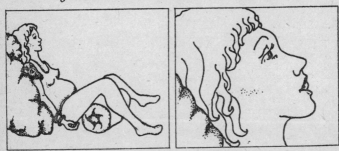

B After about 4 breaths in level A, move up to B. For this you breathe in and out through your mouth to the level of the lower ribcage with the tip of the tongue resting on the roof of your mouth, ensuring that lips are soft and open.

3. *Longer and stronger contractions—shallow breathing*

Start in level A breathing, go up to B and then up to C for the duration of one minute.
Go through it like this: conductor says, 'Contraction starts now'
after three breaths in level A, says: 'Contraction starts now'
after three breaths in level B, say: 'Getting stronger'
after fifteen seconds in level C, say: 'Getting weaker'
after three breaths in level B, say: 'Getting weaker'
after three breaths in level A, say: 'It's gone'
one deep breath and then about five to six minutes rest in between.

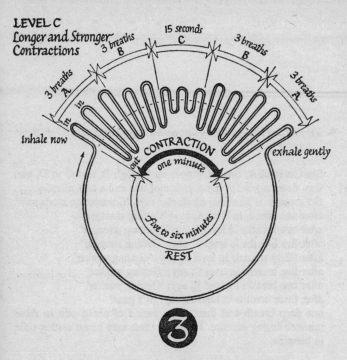

3 breaths
B

15 seconds
C

3 breaths
B

3 breaths
A

3 breaths
A

inhale now

in   in

out

CONTRACTION
one minute

exhale gently

Five to six minutes

REST

③

SHALLOW BREATHING

For use as contractions become more intense during the dilation of the cervix.

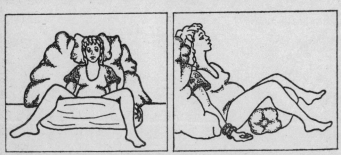

C Move up from level A, through B to C. For this depth you breathe in to breast level. As you exhale push breath out through the mouth, saying "hout".

4. *Very strong contractions—distraction technique, song and rhythmic tapping*

Start in level A, breathing goes up through B, and C to D, and then down again for the duration of one and a half minutes.
Go through it like this: conductor says, 'Contraction starts now'
after one breath in level A, say: 'Getting stronger'
after two breaths in level B, say: 'Getting stronger'
after five breaths in level C, say: 'Getting stronger'
after thirty seconds in level D, say: 'Getting weaker'
after five breaths in level C, say: 'Getting weaker'
after two breaths in level B, say: 'Getting weaker'
after three breaths in level A, say: 'It's gone'
one deep breath and then a rest period of about one to three minutes during practice. In labour there may be no resting time in between.

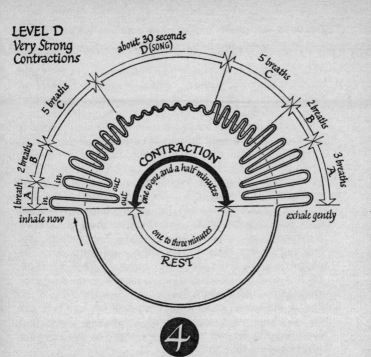

LEVEL D
Very Strong
Contractions

about 30 seconds
D (SONG)

5 breaths
C

5 breaths
C

2 breaths
B

2 breaths
B

3 breaths
A

1 breath
A

in
in

in

out

out

CONTRACTION
one to one and a half minutes

inhale now

exhale gently

one to three minutes

REST

④

DISTRACTION TECHNIQUE
(SONG)

For strongest contractions of the first stage of labour. The cervix is
approaching full dilation.

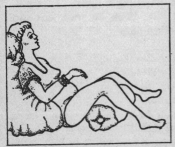 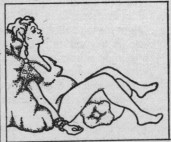

D Move up gradually from level A. After five breaths in level C, start
mouthing the song and tapping the rhythm with your finger-tips.
After about 30 seconds move down into level C, B, then A.

5. Transition—overcoming the urge to push too early: deflation technique 'Blow, one, two, one, two'

At this point, when you are not allowed to push, but must hold back, you let out air because you need, literally, to be *unable* to push. Start the practice supported as you were for the first four levels of breathing, but a little more upright, with your back straight and weight on your haunches so your physical position is not encouraging the baby to come out as it has before.

When conductor says: 'Contraction starts now' mothers should go from one breath in level B, two breaths in level C, to five seconds of the song in level D. Then the conductor should say 'Blow'. The moment of 'Blow' is the moment when the chest should sag so that the mother's diaphragm is completely relaxed. At the same time her mouth should be in the shape of an 'O' to let the surplus air escape in a kind of whistle. The conductor says 'One' and mothers bring the chest into an upright position and will feel themselves taking in air quite naturally. Then mouth the 'one two, one two' while breathing in, timed with the conductor saying it aloud. Remember to let the chest sag while saying 'blow' with the out-breath, and straighten up with the 'one two, one two'; this helps you to inhale enough for the next blowing out action. Tapping the 'one two, one two', with your hand on your knee, helps keep the rhythm.

The sagging of the chest with the gentle blowing out of surplus air is a substitute response to the push signal you are getting from your body in labour.

Go through it like this: conductor says, 'Contraction starts now'
after one breath in level B, say: 'Getting stronger'
after two breaths in level C, say: 'Getting stronger'
after five seconds in level D, say: 'Blow one two, one two'
'Blow one two, one two', repeat ten times
say 'Getting weaker'
after eight breaths in level C, say: 'Weaker still'
after four breaths in level B, say 'Weaker still'
after five breaths in level A, say: 'It's gone'
give one deep cleansing breath and
rest for approximately one minute before starting again. (During labour itself there could be more time in between contractions, or no time at all for a resting breath; it is as well to practise both.)

Overcoming the urge to push too early

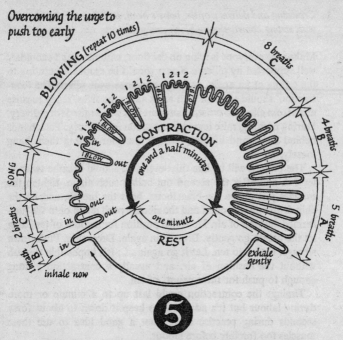

BLOWING (repeat 10 times)

1 2 1 2 · 1 2 1 2 · 1 2 1 2 · BLOW · BLOW · BLOW

1 2 1 2
in
BLOW
out

in out
in out
in

inhale now

CONTRACTION
one and a half minutes

REST
one minute

exhale gently

8 breaths
C

4 breaths
B

5 breaths
A

SONG
D

2 breaths
C

1 breath
B

5

DEFLATION TECHNIQUE
(BLOW one, two, one, two)

For use during transition. You want to push as you feel the uterus preparing to expel the baby, but should not yet, as the cervix is not fully dilated.

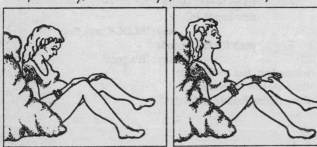

After using the song in level D you should suddenly BLOW letting the chest sag so the diaphragm is completely relaxed. Let surplus air escape. As you say ONE, bring your head up. Air is inhaled naturally as you say TWO, ONE, TWO. Then BLOW for the exhalation, letting the chest sag again.

6. *Crowning and delivery of the baby's head: utilizing the urge to push with strong contractions—block and push*

Make sure everyone is lying on the floor, with head and shoulders well supported by pillows. Knees should be crooked, pointing to the ceiling at an angle, and legs of course wide apart. The 'contraction' should start off with arms along the sides, ready to raise arms from elbow to wrist, to support legs when raised for delivery. During pushing, raise legs in preparation for delivery. Tuck hands behind knees and lift feet just off the floor, letting them hang loosely.

The pattern will be like this: everyone should breathe twice in level A and after the second out-breath suck air in, tighten the muscles just above the breastbone, hold the breath, and let the chin drop onto the chest and the ribcage push down onto the just-formed cushion of air. Hold this position for a count of ten, then let the breath go gently. Breathe in again. Drop chin. Push down ribcage. Count to ten. Let it go again . . . It's impossible to push without the cushion of air, and usually a contraction is long enough to push for three counts of ten.

Timing: the contraction could last up to a minute or more during labour but it's advisable to keep it down to about forty seconds during practice as it's not a good idea to use these muscles too forcibly before labour.

Go through it like this: conductor says: 'Contraction starts now' after two breaths in level A, say: 'Legs in position'
at third 'in' breath,   say: 'BLOCK and push'
        push for ten seconds
        let go breath gently
        new breath in
                say: 'BLOCK and push'
        push for ten seconds
                say: 'It's gone'
release legs, feet to the floor
three breaths in level C
three resting breaths in level A

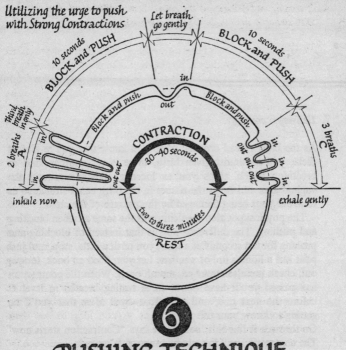

Utilizing the urge to push with Strong Contractions

Let breath go gently

10 seconds BLOCK and PUSH

10 seconds BLOCK and PUSH

in

Block and push

out

Block and push

Think breath in ply

2 breaths A

in in

in in

CONTRACTION
30-40 seconds

out out

out out in in

3 breaths C

inhale now

two to three minutes

exhale gently

REST

6
PUSHING TECHNIQUE
(BLOCK and PUSH)

This is for pushing with strong contractions that accompany the bearing-down sensation. Dilation of the cervix is complete and the baby's head is ready to crown for delivery.

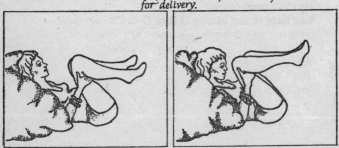

Raise your legs in a comfortable position. Let breathing move up until the urge to push overtakes you, then inhale, hold the breath, BLOCK IT, and PUSH hard with the peak of the contraction.

7. *Delivery: 'panting'*

As the baby's head crowns, when you know that you're almost there, you've almost given birth, there is yet another kind of breathing which keeps you as loose as possible around the vaginal area and helps the tissues in the birth canal stretch so as to avoid your being damaged by the passage of the child.

The physical position for delivery is the same as when blocking and pushing. The difference now is that instead of blocking and pushing for ten seconds at a time, you push a little, stop, and just pant like a lioness in hot weather. Let your head go back, tongue out, cheek muscles stretched, mouth open. When the contraction has passed you'll have about three resting breaths in level C before the next one, and after that—well after that you'll be getting to know your offspring.

Go through it like this: conductor says, 'Contraction starts now'
The contraction will last about twenty-five seconds
one breath in
block and push for a few seconds
say: 'stop pushing'
    'pant like a lioness' for about twenty seconds
say: 'It's over'
take three resting breaths in level C

Panting for delivery

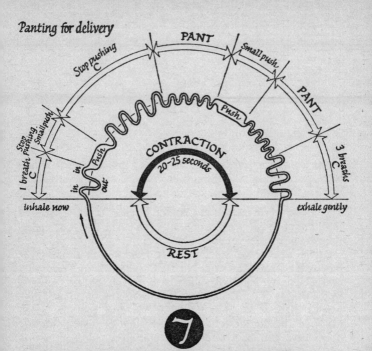

PANT

Stop pushing
C

Small push

PANT

Stop pushing
Small push

1 breath
Stop pushing
C

3 breaths
C

in
in
Push
out

Push

CONTRACTION
20-25 seconds

inhale now

exhale gently

REST

7

DELIVERY TECHNIQUE
(PANTING)

For use as the baby's head crowns and the child is being delivered.

FRONT DELIVERY

SIDE DELIVERY

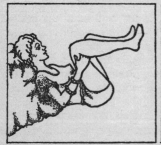

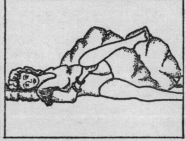

Hold your legs in the same position as for pushing, but simply pant, like a lioness in the hot sun, as you feel the uterus gathering itself up to expel the baby completely.

APPENDIX II

Legal Notes

In a case where medical or obstetric practices in a pregnancy or labour result in the maiming or death of an infant, the legal implications are now under consideration.

At the time of writing the Law Commission in England has published a report (Law Com. No. 60, Cmnd 5709) which deals with civil liabilities for injuries to unborn children. This has been provoked by the tragedy of the Thalidomide children and the question of their parents' right to compensation from the drug company which marketed Thalidomide as harmless medication for pregnant women. There have also been cases where premature induction or unnecessary medical interference has caused death or brain damage in an unborn child. Many of these cases have yet to be settled definitively. The Law Commission's paper covers any situation in which an arbitrary medical decision leads to injury or death in the womb, so that the injured child has legal cause for action against the person who injured him.

In the case of the Thalidomide children settlement was finally negotiated after protracted legal battles, in the spring of 1975. This clearly upheld the right of action for the unborn child in that children maimed in the womb are now legally bound to receive compensation. There is now a Private Members Bill going before Parliament which legislates further to safeguard the rights of the unborn child.

The aborted or stillborn child has no rights, although parents can claim funeral expenses in the event of proved negligence. However, any child brought living into the world after an attempted abortion is entitled to claim against any negligent party. Out of 400,000 abortions in New York, for instance, two children survived the ordeal to be born after a full term of gestation in the womb. One was seriously handicapped. Now the handicapped child has the right to sue the abortionist.

In 1968, Dr G. S. Dawes' remarks about the independence of the fetus from the mother was one of the first voiced medical opinions that three years later was to lead to a court ruling in Melbourne, Australia, that a baby injured in its mother's womb is entitled to damages.

Dr Dawes, of the Nuffield Institute for Medical Research, Oxford, said in a summing-up address to a symposium of doctors involved in fetal medicine, that:

'Most of the papers in this symposium . . . have emphasized to a greater extent the relative independence of the embryo or fetus from its mother.'

The Melbourne ruling was the first time a court anywhere has spelled out the rights of an unborn child. Still most doctors are careful to clarify that in their opinion the fetus does not 'become a person' until it reaches twenty-eight weeks gestation; it is not normally capable of independent life until then.

Family-Centred Maternity Care

The most radical and far-reaching changes in hospital maternity care on both sides of the Atlantic have resulted from intense struggle around the institutions themselves and the laws that control them. The setting up of family-centred maternity care, which permits parents to share the childbearing experience and have access to their baby immediately after birth, allows mother and child to leave hospital within twelve hours of the birth, so deepening the welcoming love relationship between woman, man and child.

In America there has been the introduction of rooming-in, the legal father of the child is allowed to share a room with his wife and child. This is one way of going halfway to meet the problem separation and disorientation after birth. In Britain this is not a practice that is generally known—neither is it realized by most women that they can in fact discharge themselves from hospital whenever they wish.

Again in America, a woman politician has taken the daring step of trying to give the biological father of the child the legal right to insist on being present at the birth of his own offspring. Congresswoman Martha Griffiths has introduced a bill (HR 1504).

The proposal is as follows:

'Whereas it is the natural human right of a woman to determine the manner of her child's birth; Whereas the participation of the father in the childbirth process undermines rigid, traditional sex roles from the beginning; Whereas it is a sexist notion that childbirth is "women's work"; it is rather a family affair . . .; Whereas there does exist a double standard in American medicine prejudicial against women: Be it resolved . . . to provide for hospitals to allow the biological father to attend the birth of his child, if the woman consents.'

Martha Griffiths is in a position and has the determination to do something about a situation most women feel deeply about, but make no move for change because they cannot draw on the knowledge of correct procedure.

APPENDIX III

Childbirth Organizations

ENGLAND: The National Childbirth Trust, No 9 Queensborough Terrace, London, W.2, is a charity run organization specializing in Education for Parenthood. From them you will find more details on the specific method of psychoprophylaxis, lectures, seminars, films on childbirth. They have preparation courses for childbirth, most of which include an evening for fathers. They hold meetings, dispense advice, sell books and very good adjustable maternity bras. Started by a mother in 1956 as an association, it became a Trust and recognized as a Charity in 1959. Now there are over five thousand members, with fifty branches in the British Isles and a hundred and fifty overseas representatives. Some branches organize babysitting, emergency help and play groups, and all are well supported by midwives, physiotherapists and workers involved in anything to do with maternity.

U.S.A.: There are several equivalent groups in America. The aims are roughly the same—relaxed natural birth and well-informed parents, but the names are different, and there are branches in different states.

American Society for Psychoprophylaxis in Obstetrics: 164 West 79th Street, New York
Long Island Chapter: 1520 Blue Spruce Street, Wantagh, New York
Los Angeles Chapter: 13231 Calcutta Street, Sylmar, California
Connecticut CALM: 38 Basyberry Lane, Westport, Connecticut
C.E.A. of Greater St Louis (Childbirth Education Association): 2 Chafford Wood, St Louis, Missouri

Salt Lake City C.E.A. (Childbirth Education Association): St Marks' Hospital, Salt Lake City, Utah

C.W.P.E.A.: 201–34 Snowden, Detroit, Michigan

Franklin County Childbirth Association: Village Green, Greenfield, Massachusetts

H.O.P.E.: 5327 Imogene Street, Houston, Texas

Lamaze Association for Childbirth Group: Ann Arbor, Michigan

Washington Area Lamaze Childbirth Group: 2610 Henderson Avenue, Heaton, Maryland

Haight Ashbury Women's Clinic: 1101 Masonic, San Francisco, California (pregnancy testing, birth control, abortion advice, health service)

Problem Pregnancy Information Center: Box 9090, Standord, California (free pregnancy counselling, adoption placement, abortion advice)

Chicago Women's Liberation Union: 852 Belmont, Chicago, Illinois; 312-348-4300

Pregnancy Counseling Service: 3 Joy Street, Boston, Massachusetts 02108; 413-732-1852

Women's Counseling Service, 621 West Lake Street, Minneapolis, Minnesota 55408; 612-827-3812

Counseling and Referral Service: Women's Center, 1824 Los Lomas, University of New Mexico, Albuquerque, New Mexico 87106; 505-277-3716

The American College of Nurse-Midwives: 48 East 92nd Street, New York, New York 10028; 212-369-7300 (this is the professional organization for nurse midwives in the United States)

There is also the Lamaze Education for Childbirth: 7 West 96th Street, New York

In New York too is the Maternity Centers Association, 48 East 92nd Street, New York, 10028 (they can provide you with a beautifully clear and well-illustrated large birth atlas, as well as information on midwives who are prepared to do home deliveries). Mrs Ruth Watson Lubic is the General Director.

The International Childbirth Education Association has as its co-presidents John and Doris Haire, 251 Nottingham Way, Hillside, New Jersey, 10205. They put out an excellent and informative journal called the *I.C.E.A. News*, which can be mailed to you on application to P.O. Box 5852, Milwaukee, Wisconsin 53220. There are regional directors in various states.

If you are interested in hospitals which encourage natural childbirth, you can also contact:

New Life Center: Doctor's Hospital, 28th and West Wells Street, Milwaukee, Wisconsin 53208; 414-344-9400

Dr Sumner, The Manchester Community Hospital, Connecticut

Here they have imported a special labour bed from Sweden that does not have the inconveniences to a woman of the usual delivery bed where she is flat on her back. There is also a special room called the 'Lamaze Room' where labour and delivery take place without the woman having to be moved in mid-labour.

Dr William Hazlett, of the Maternity Hospital in Nesbitt, Pennsylvania, actually teaches husbands to deliver their children and takes photographers into the labour room.

APPENDIX IV

Information for Home Deliveries

If you are interested in having your baby at home, or at least finding out about how you should go about it, who could attend you, and whether there is any reason for taking extra care in your particular case because of possible obstetrical complications, here is a list of organizations to contact for information. You can also try your regional branch of any natural or psychoprophylaxis childbirth organization.

In England you can contact the Royal College of Midwives to find the name and address of a midwife to attend you at home, and to bring you up to date with exactly what a midwife can and cannot do. The International Confederation of Midwives in Oxford Street, London, W.1, will provide the same service, and they also know details applicable to other countries.

In America you can write to the International Childbirth Education Association at P.O. Box 5852, Milwaukee, Wisconsin 53220, or The Maternity Centers Association, 48 East 92nd Street, New York, 10028. The American Society for Psychoprophylaxis in Obstetrics, Inc., will also provide you with information wherever you are; contact: 1523 L Street NW, Suite 410, Washington DC, 20005.

If you live in California and want guidance for home birth there are several groups to approach:

The University of California Child Care Division
The Florence Nightingale Birth Collective
The Commune Health Education Project (developed at the University of California Medical Center)

There are also nurse-midwife training programmes in Los Angeles, Loma Linda and San Francisco.

There are several male doctors in California who have pioneered home delivery and have dropped out of the hospital system to provide for women wanting home births:

Michael Witt, M.D., a general practitioner from Port Reyes, California, who works with Dr Wes Sokoloski in community medical practice which includes home birth; also

Jeff Anderson, M.D., who practises in Mill Valley, Marin County, California.

APPENDIX V

Homoeopathic Stockists and Herbal Supply Houses

If you want to know more about homoeopathy, or to contact your nearest homoeopathic doctor, you can get in touch with the British Homoeopathic Association, 27a Devonshire Street, London, W.1. In London there is an excellent chemist with a comprehensive stock of homoeopathic goods called: A. Nelson & Company, Duke Street, London, W.1. Information in the United States can be obtained from: The American Institute of Homoeopathy, Suite 506, 6231 Leesburg Pike, Falls Church, Va. 22044.

Herbal Supply Houses in the United Kingdom

Baldwins, 173 Walworth Road, London, S.E.7 (they keep between 300 and 400 loose herbs)

Crittens, 39 Park Road, London, N.8 (they stock about 150 different kinds of herbs)

Falcon Herbal and Health Food Stores, 44 Falcon Road, London, S.W.11 (they also stock about 150 different herbs)

Culpeper House (main branch), Bruton Street, London, W.1

As with homoeopathy, it is always wiser to follow the guidance of the qualified. If you want treatment with a qualified medical herbalist, and you live in England, you can trace one through the Secretary of the National Institute of Medical Herbalists at:

68 London Road, Leicester, England
and the Secretary of the Society of Herbalists, at 34 Boscobel Place, London, S.W.1

Herbal Supply Houses in the U.S.A.

The Herb Society of America, 300 Massachusetts Avenue, Boston, Massachusetts 12115, U.S.A.
Nature's Herb Company, 281 Ellis Street, San Francisco, California
Indiana Botanic Gardens, Hammon, Indiana 46325
Aphrodisia, 28 Carmine Street, New York City, New York 10014
Kiehl's Pharmacy, 109 3rd Avenue, New York City, New York 10003
Nichol's Garden Nursery, 1190 North Pacific Highway, Albany, Oregon
Penn Herb Company, 603 North Second Street, Philadelphia, Pennsylvania
Meadowbrook Herb Garden, Wyoming, Rhode Island

In Canada

Worldwide Herb Limited, 11 St Catherine Street East, Montreal 129

APPENDIX VI

Suggested Reading

Birth

Awake and Aware by Irwin Chabon, M.D., Delacorte, New York 1969

Birth by Caterine Milinaire, Harmony, New York 1974

Birth by David Metzner, Ballantine, New York 1973

Childbirth without Fear by Dr Grantly Dick-Read, Heinemann Medical, London 1942, 5th edition revised 1968; Harper & Row, New York 1970

Childbirth without Violence by Dr Frederick Leboyer, Wildwood House, London 1975; Alfred Knopf, New York 1975

The Cultural Warping of Childbirth by Doris and John Haire, I.C.E.A., New Jersey, U.S.A. 1972

Everywoman: A Gynaecological Guide for Life by Derek Llewellyn Jones, M.D., Faber, London 1975; Harper & Row, New York 1970

The Experience of Childbirth by Sheila Kitzinger, Gollancz, London 1962; Taplinger, New York 1972; Penguin Books, Harmondsworth 1967 (4th edition 1978)

Husband-Coached Childbirth by Robert Bradley, M.D., New York 1965

Immaculate Deception by Suzanne Arms, Houghton Mifflin, Boston 1975

Natural Childbirth by Dr Grantly Dick-Read, Heinemann, London 1933

The New Childbirth by Erna Wright, Tandem, London 1964; Pocket Books, New York 1971

Our Bodies Ourselves by the Boston Women's Book Collective, Simon & Schuster, New York 1972

Pregnancy by Gordon Bourne, F.R.C.S., F.R.C.O.G., Cassell, London 1972, Pan revised edition 1975; Harper & Row, New York 1974

Pregnancy and Birth by Alan F. Guttmacher, M.D., Signet Books, New York 1971

Pregnancy, Birth and Family Planning: A Guide for Expectant Parents in the 1970s by Alan F. Guttmacher, M.D., Viking Press, New York 1973

A Season to be Born by Suzanne and John Arms, Harper & Row, New York 1973

Six Practical Lessons for an Easier Childbirth by Elisabeth Bing, Bantam, New York 1969

Homoeopathy

*Homoeopathic Drug Pictures by M. L. Tyler, M.D., L.R.C.R., L.R.F.P.S., L.R.C.S., Health Science Press, Sussex 1942

*Homoeopathic Materia Medica by William Boericke, M.D., Boericke & Tafel, U.S.A.

*Homoeopathy by G. Ruthven Mitchell, W. H. Allen, London 1975

Homoeopathy by George Vithoulkas, Avon, New York 1972

*Homoeopathy for Mother and Infant by Douglas M. Borland, M.D., British Homoeopathic Association

*Children's Types by Douglas Borland, M.B., F.F.Hom., British Homoeopathic Association

*Elements of Homoeopathy by D. M. Gibson, M.B., F.R.C.S.(Edin), F.F.Hom., British Homoeopathic Association

*First Aid Homoeopathy in Accidents and Ailments by D. M. Gibson, M.B., F.R.C.S.(Edin), F.F.Hom., British Homoeopathic Association

*Homoeopathic Medicine by Harris L. Coulter, American Institute of Homoeopathy

Homoeopathy in America: the Rise and Fall of a Medical Heresy by Martin Kaufman, Johns Hopkins University Press, Baltimore 1971

The Patient Not the Cure by Dr Margery Blackie, MacDonald & Janes, London 1976

* *Note:* These books are available in both the U.S.A. and the U.K., through specialist bookshops and the relevant organizations.

Herbal Medicine

Culpeper's Complete Herbal by Dr Nicholas Culpeper, M.D., written in 1653 and first published by Thomas Kelly, London; a new edition is now available by W. Foulsham & Co., London; Sterling, New York 1959

The Herbalist by Joseph E. Meyer, Sterling, New York 1968

Manual of Nutrition by Ministry of Agriculture, Fisheries and Food, London, 1970. Available from Her Majesty's Stationery Offices. (London address: 49 High Holborn, London)

A Pattern of Herbs by Meg Rutherford, with a section on Herbal Medicine by Ann Warren-Davis, M.N.I.M.H., George Allen and Unwin, London 1975; Doubleday, U.S.A. 1976

Your Daily Food: Recipe for Survival by Doris Grant. Faber and Faber, London, 1973

Index

MORE ABOUT PENGUINS
AND PELICANS

Penguinews, which appears every month, contains details of all the new books issued by Penguins as they are published. From time to time it is supplemented by our stocklist which includes around 5,000 titles.

A specimen copy of *Penguinews* will be sent to you free on request. Please write to Dept EP, Penguin Books Ltd, Harmondsworth, Middlesex, for your copy.

In the U.S.A.: For a complete list of books available from Penguins in the United States write to Dept CS, Penguin Books, 625 Madison Avenue, New York, New York 10022.

In Canada: For a complete list of books available from Penguins in Canada write to Penguin Books Canada Ltd, 2801 John Street, Markham, Ontario L3R 1B4.